THE

Living Beauty
Detox Program

THE
Living Beauty
Detox Program

The Revolutionary Diet
for Each and Every Season
of a Woman's Life

A<small>NN</small> L<small>OUISE</small> G<small>ITTLEMAN</small>, M.S, C.N.S.

with Ann Castro

HarperSanFrancisco
A Division of HarperCollinsPublishers

This book will educate the reader about natural drugs, remedies, treatments, medicines, and "dietary supplements." It is based on the research and experience of the author, who is a licensed nutritionist. This is not meant to be a substitute for medical attention. Rather, readers with specific medical concerns or symptoms should seek advice from a physician. Every effort has been made to ensure that the selections of natural drugs, remedies, treatments, medicines, cures, dietary supplements, and applicable dosages are in accordance with current recommendations and practices. But because research in these areas is ongoing, the reader is always cautioned to check with a health professional about specific recommendations.

HarperCollins books may be purchased for educational, business, or sales promotional use. For information please write: Special Markets Department, HarperCollins Publishers Inc., 10 East 53rd Street, New York, NY 10022.

HarperCollins Web site: http://www.harpercollins.com

HarperCollins®, ♨®, and HarperSanFrancisco™ are trademarks of HarperCollins Publishers Inc.

FIRST HARPERCOLLINS PAPERBACK EDITION PUBLISHED IN 2001

Designed by Jessica Shatan

Library of Congress Cataloging-in-Publication Data

Gittleman, Ann Louise
    The living beauty detox program: the revolutionary diet for each and every season of a woman's life: eat right to cleanse yourself of toxins, manage your hormones, and bring out your best looks/Ann Louise Gittleman with Ann Castro.—1st ed.
      p. cm.
    Includes bibliographical references and index.
    ISBN 0-06-251627-2 (cloth)
    ISBN 0-06-251628-0 (pbk.)
    1. Nutrition. 2. Detoxification (health) 3. Beauty, Personal. 4. Women—Health and hygiene. I. Castro, Ann. II. Title
    RA784.G537 2000
    613.2—dc21   99–043044

01 02 03 04 05 ❖/HADD 10 9 8 7 6 5 4 3 2 1

*This book is dedicated to women everywhere,
but especially to the Baby Boomers
who are revolutionizing concepts of
aging, beauty, and detoxification*

Contents

Acknowledgments ix

Introduction 1

1 | Turning Beauty Inside Out 5

2 | The Road to Ruin Is Paved with Good Intentions 13

3 | Seasonal Beauty: Internal Cleansing and Support for Spring, Summer, Fall, Winter 27

4 | Spring Seasonal Detox Diet 49

5 | Summer Seasonal Detox Diet 62

6 | Autumn Seasonal Detox Diet 78

7 | Winter Seasonal Detox Diet 95

8 | Beauty Routines for Ages and Stages 108

9 | Detoxing the Inner 147

10 | Detoxing the Outer 162

11 | Living Beauty Alphabet of Vitamins and Minerals 177

Appendix: The Two-Week Fat Flush 203

Selected References 211

Resources 221

Index 235

Acknowledgments

I am most grateful to a rather unique cast of characters whose unwavering support and talent transformed my musings into a manuscript.

To Liz Perle—my HarperSanFrancisco Editor-at-Large—who brilliantly nurtured my *Living Beauty* concept in the first place. Thank you, Liz, for your encouragement, direction, and belief in this project.

To David Hennessy—Associate Editor—who was always there when I needed him and helped me in so many ways.

To Ann Castro—who embraced the magic of *Living Beauty* with creative passion, patience, and perseverance. My most heartfelt thanks for your assisting me in translating my tapes and thoughts and reflecting them so beautifully on the printed page of this manuscript.

To the entire HarperSanFrancisco staff—including Diane Gedymin, Margery Buchanan, Amy Durgan, Meg Lenihan, Steve Hanselman, Susan Naythons, Lisa Zuniga, and Terri Leonard—who have become my literary family.

To the staff at Les Nouvelles Esthetiques—especially David Friedman, Monica Schuloff, and Joel Gerson, who introduced my work to the beauty industry through their trade shows.

To Dr. Howard Murad—CEO/Founder Murad, Inc.—who graciously allowed me to speak at his special international conferences.

To Sondra Metzger—that unforgettable redhead whom I met in Palm Springs who shared many of her time-tested beauty secrets—thanks to the referral of Susan Meredith, an unforgettable brunette beauty!

To my precious mentors—who have passed on but left behind a body of work that still inspires me and nourishes my nutritional soul—Dr. Hazell Parcells, Gayelord Hauser, Linda Clark, Carl Pfeiffer, Paul Eck, Hanna Kroeger, and Nathan Pritikin.

To the beauty care professionals who have been instrumental in my own journey to Living Beauty—to Anna Hugdahl from Santa Fe, New Mexico, you are my French treasure . . . to Julie Bethke from San Francisco, California, Julie—I adore you . . . to Mary The from San Francisco, a marvelous role model for the entire cosmetic industry and a true renaissance woman and wonderful new friend . . . to Mary Ann Alexander from Bozeman, Montana, who always managed to fit me in and helped me look my Living Beauty best . . . to JoAnne Findorak from Mill Valley, California, who has been a true friend since those early days in the Village and is now a Living Beauty expert!

To the nutritionists and doctors whom I truly respect as professionals and like as people—Dr. Nan Katherine Fuchs, Dr. Hyla Cass, Susun Weed, Dr. Tori Hudson, and Cheryl Townsley. Thank you for all the wonderful work you are doing far and wide in your unique and special ways.

To Maria Low—for helping to keep a semblace of order in my personal life day in and day out. Maria is an angel.

To Dr. Ron Davis—for his expertise in Chinese Medicine and his ability to needle me in the right places.

To Claudia Krevat—for helping me maintain my Living Beauty diet plan through her extraordinary cooking talents.

To Stuart Gittleman—beloved brother, Operations Manager of ALG, Inc., and my right hand twenty-four hours a day, seven days a week, 365 days a year. Stu, you were such a calming influence in the midst of "the white tornado," providing invaluable research assistance and attending to oh-so-many details throughout the writing of this book (sorry ladies . . . he *is* married with two lovely children).

To James William Templeton—who has become my anchor and my rock through creative chaos and all the good times. James, forever is as far as I'll go.

THE
Living Beauty Detox Program

Introduction

All seasons of life are beautiful. Aging is a problem only when you
stop liking yourself as a person. Fortunately, I still like myself inside
and out. Not in a vain way—I just feel good in my skin.
SOPHIA LOREN,
Women and Beauty

When Estée Lauder launched a new product targeting women in their
forties, fifties, and sixties, they asked me to join their professional panel
of experts for a press conference in New York City to discuss the nutritional needs of the changing woman. I was speaking on how eating the
right kind and amounts of fats, proteins, and carbohydrates could
increase vitality and bring out our vibrant beauty. And that's where the
idea for this book was born. As I looked out at all the young faces in the
audience, I couldn't help but wish I knew at their age what I do now:
protecting our beauty begins in our youth and continues throughout
every age and stage of life. This book is for mothers and their daugh-
ters—and women of all ages—who want to discover, awaken, and pre-
serve the unique beauty living within them—the lifelong beauty, the
living beauty, that only good nutrition and tender care can produce.
   Many cosmetic companies are starting to address the various ages and
stages of a woman's life. Even women's magazines have been horning in
on this trend, targeting women not only in their teens and twenties, but

also in the prime of life at thirty, forty, fifty, and beyond. Although this is a noble effort, I can't see that much has really changed. Sure, many companies in the beauty industry are finally regarding products as treatments and formulating them with the same beautifying antioxidants we should normally be ingesting in foods and supplements, like vitamins A, C, and E. But when I sat on that panel in New York and noticed an abundance of popcorn and candy being served among the refreshments, I knew the great beauty cover-up was still alive and well. The cold, hard fact is that we're all under the mistaken impression that beauty still comes from the outside and can only be purchased in a jar. Like magic, the right cosmetic "eliminates" crow's feet, "creates" glowing skin, "strengthens" nails, "softens" hair, and even makes cellulite disappear. But when you remove the cover-up, what do you have? A heavy dose of reality. Take it from me, camouflage isn't the answer. The right nutrition, internal cleansing, and hormonal harmony are the pathways to attaining natural beauty and vitality. You can empower yourself to achieve those goals by following the Living Beauty plan as well as the many suggestions I've described throughout this book.

The bottom line is we all want to look good no matter what age or stage of life we're in—a youthful twenty-something or a vibrant sixtyish. In fact, while I was on the panel, I had the wonderful opportunity to meet Karen Graham, a legendary model from the seventies whom Estée Lauder decided to use for its new product campaign. Karen, well known a little over two decades ago as *Vogue*'s cover girl, made a statement that I believe captured the way most of us feel: "Women my age should feel great about themselves. . . . I think it's important to get the message out there that we're vital, active, important, and beautiful." I couldn't agree more. Like many other women in the baby-boomer generation, I don't mind looking good for my age, I just don't want to look older than I am.

We feel better when we look our best, and, let's face it, looking good gets you places in our extremely visual society. Just ask psychologist and researcher Nancy Etcoff, author of *Survival of the Prettiest: The Science of Beauty* (1999). Etcoff discovered some revealing facts about our fascination with beauty. Three-month-old babies typically stared longer at the same kind of faces adults find most appealing. And good-looking people appear to be way ahead of the game from the beginning of infancy onward; mothers played with pretty babies more than home-lier ones; unattractive children were more likely to be abused; teachers expected better-looking students to be smarter; and law enforcement officials (including judges and juries) tend to ease up on the nicer-looking sector of society. All of this has prompted Etcoff to believe we are born with "beauty detectors," which cause us to be attracted to indi-viduals who symbolize physical beauty, like Cindy Crawford, Naomi Campbell, and the legendary Marilyn Monroe.

Are we born with beauty detectors? Well, the quest for beauty has certainly spanned the history of humanity. Forty thousand years ago people painted their faces with red ocher crayons to look attractive. Around the time of Mesolithic Era (10,000 years B.C.E.) castor oil and animal grease were the in thing for softening skin. Lipsticks were a hot item 5,000 years ago in Ur. And beauty seekers in 1000 B.C.E. kept their bodies silky smooth with scrubs made out of clay and sand. Cleopatra, Queen of the Nile—a name we all equate with alluring beauty—kept herself looking good for Mark Antony by placing sesame seed and barley packs on her face. Greek physicians created the first cold creams out of beeswax, olive oil, and rose water, while Romans poured beautifying milk from goats and asses into their communal baths. Vigilant beauty buffs, the Venetians dyed their hair with plant color, then covered it with clay and baked in the sun. Even monks in Florence during the 1500s got in on the act, establishing the first per-fumery. And on and on it continued right up to our modern-day breast implants, face-lifts, and liposuction, which could be mere reflections of that age-old pattern Etcoff refers to.

Or maybe it's something more. Thanks to the powerful media-driven advertising machine, we've been hurled into the fantasy world of computer-enhanced photography and unrealistic expectations. In fact, a psychological study done on women found that after spending just three minutes looking at models in a fashion magazine, 70 percent of the female participants felt depressed, guilty, and shameful. Comparing themselves to airbrushed images, these women saw themselves as inad-equate, not measuring up to that perfect ten on the beauty scale. But who really does? The truth is the models don't even look like that! All too often in today's society, women are developing self-esteem issues as they strive for the unattainable instead of feeling free to discover their individual authenticity. The result? Bulimia, anorexia, and compulsive overeating disorders as well as the many health risks that go along with them.

Since the media propels these ideals, it's not surprising that most of the women suffering from eating disorders are between the ages of fourteen and twenty-five. These impressionable young women are willing to pay any price to be thin and look like the models or actresses they idolize. When *People* magazine in April of 1999 surveyed 490 of the country's largest colleges and universities, they discovered most female students were willing to continue their eating disorders "as long as guys desired them, girlfriends envied them, and society spurred them on regardless of the physical consequence to their bodies." What it all boils down to is these young women actually believe they are ugly because of the beauty lies they've been told on TV, in the movies, and in magazines. I wonder if they know that sex symbol Marilyn Monroe— still regarded as "hot" by men of all ages today—was a size twelve!

As you can see, our understanding and values of beauty are extremely distorted, which is why I felt compelled to write this book. My hope is that you not only will see and believe in the reality of your own unique brand of both outer and inner beauty, but that you also will be inspired to take charge of your body, mind, and spirit using the life-changing regimens and tips I've outlined. For the woman in her teens and twenties, this book can help lay a firm foundation for individual beauty that will last a lifetime. The thirty- or forty-something woman can learn how to revitalize and maintain a youthful appearance throughout those not-so-distant menopausal years. And women who are fifty and beyond can discover how to rejuvenate their looks to enjoy a timeless beauty and put the zest back into their life.

A youthful glow, skin that's soft to the touch, luster-rich hair, strong healthy nails, a serene spirit, and a nourished soul: true beauty is here for each of us no matter what our age. It's only a matter of understanding how to create it. As you seek to uncover your living beauty, may this book empower you to soar to new heights of joy, self-confidence, and love.

1

Turning Beauty Inside Out

You really *can* be beautifully transformed and unlock your individual potential. And you don't have to have those illusory perfect-ten features to do it, either. Just by following the Living Beauty regimen in this book, true beauty is just weeks away. No kidding. You'll actually start to see improvements in those troublesome ailments you've been fighting, whether it's cracks around your mouth, a pimply face, a sallow complexion, thinning hair, premature wrinkling, blotchy skin, fatty deposits like cellulite, splitting nails, soft bones, or even unhealthy gums that are ruining your smile. The key to developing a beautiful physical appearance is to start from the inside out by clearing away physical and emotional toxins. Simply slapping on moisturizers and cover-ups just won't do it anymore, especially with the overload of waste materials and poisons inundating all of us in this new millennium. The truth is, in today's toxic world you have to go deeper to create total beauty, which means properly cleansing your body on all levels. Which is why detoxifying your system has never been more important or more urgent to your overall well-being and looks.

That's where this book promises help. Filled with cutting-edge science, ancient wisdom, and common sense, it will show you how to turn your present approach to beauty and health around—or rather, inside out.

You'll begin by starting fresh with a clean slate, cleansing your way to beauty with a clear-cut detox diet plan designed in harmony with nature's seasons. Both the Living Beauty Detox Diets and the maintenance program (which you can alter to suit your individual needs) include beauty-building foods, herbs, spices, and essential fatty acids to help repair, strengthen, and invigorate cells so you have a rejuvenated, youthful glow. Then to further enhance your newly acquired radiant looks, you'll also find a number of natural beauty tips and routines that have been specifically designed for your special concerns during your particular stage of life. You'll also discover ways to take your quest for beauty to higher ground, because beauty goes far beyond the physical. I've found that beauty actually emanates from your spiritual, emotional, and mental being, so I've included some innovative methods to help you remove the "inner" toxins from your deepest self. In addition, you'll learn how to identify and protect yourself from unsuspected "outer" toxins that lurk about in your home surroundings and thwart your beauty on a daily basis. Finally, we'll wrap it up with a review of the Living Beauty Alphabet of Vitamins and Minerals, showing where they are found and what is the optimum beauty dosage that will help you sustain your new beauty foundation and continue to secure younger-looking skin, silky hair, strong nails, and a trimmer body. As you embark on this journey to create a more glorious, beautiful image inside and out, you can be sure of one thing: you'll be enveloped in a joyous and rewarding experience of self-discovery that will undoubtedly transcend the media-manufactured beauty values you once held so dear.

The Living Beauty Mainstays

When you are feeling your best, you look your best. In fact, unless you are nutritionally supported from within, it is virtually impossible to look really good because real beauty isn't just skin-deep. Beauty isn't about how thin you are, about smearing some cover-up on your face, or even about wearing the right kind of lipstick. Achieving true beauty—even in our media-swayed, visual society—begins by turning things inside out. Here are the dynamic seven beauty fundamentals every woman needs in her life.

- a cleansed, detoxed system

- purified water

- powerful proteins

- beautifying oils

- energizing, immune-boosting veggies and fruits

- revitalizing vitamins, minerals, and antioxidants

- balanced hormones

When you look in the mirror and notice beauty problems—dull, grayish skin, brittle hair from hell, and thin, splitting nails—you're actually seeing outward reflections of inner imbalances caused not only by a lack of the vital Living Beauty essentials mentioned above, but also by toxic overload and mental, emotional, or spiritual blocks. These beauty thieves manifest themselves throughout the different ages and stages of our lives and are heightened by everyday stress and natural hormonal shifts. Let's take a closer look at each one.

Toxic Overload: Beautify Your System

Beautiful definitely begins by detoxifying your body. It is *the* first step toward a healthier, more radiant you. After all, every day you're immersed in a chemical war—outside and inside your body. A sea of toxins surrounds you, from environmental chemicals in solvents, plastics, and adhesives to poisons in makeup, moisturizers, nail polish, hair dyes, and shampoos. Even food and soil are inundated with pesticides and herbicides, not to mention the contaminants and parasites lurking in water. Everything you touch, taste, breathe, and eat is propelling the leading engine of the detoxification process, your liver, into overdrive. And once your liver becomes overwhelmed by all the poisons it has to neutralize, transform, or process, it loses its ability to function properly. This in turn leads to a cascade of disastrous health consequences and causes vital body systems to malfunction—as well as the quality of your beauty to suffer.

A lean, mean, chemical-clearing machine, the liver cleans one and one-half quarts of blood every minute of the day so that other organs can be nourished by purified blood, and it neutralizes toxic wastes, sending them off to the next detox organ, the kidneys, for elimination. The liver also chemically deactivates vital hormones (such as estrogen), thereby maintaining hormonal balance, sustains the body's major detoxification pathways, makes bile salts, produces cholesterol and amino acids, stores vitamin A, D, B_{12}, and iron, metabolizes fat for energy, and regulates blood sugar for energy. Alcohol, prescription or over-the-counter drugs, fatty foods, smoking, and a plethora of environmental toxins (from pesticides and exhaust fumes to hair spray and gasoline) thwart the work of this blockbuster workaholic.

If toxins, rancid fats, or drugs clog up the liver's detoxification pathways, secondary symptoms will arise. Blood sugar levels fluctuate, and chronic fatigue and PMS or perimenopausal problems such as bloating, anxiety, and irritability manifest. And when the liver is congested, it presses on the vein that connects it to the colon (the portal vein) and causes hemorrhoids, sometimes referred to as the "varicose veins" of the colon. If toxins run rampant, the body chooses to store them in fatty tissues (which are metabolically less active than other tissues), where they can stay for years!

When your liver is on overload, toxins find their way through your skin, and radically affect its clarity and elasticity. The skin, like the liver, is a major detoxifying organ, so waste materials exit through the skin's pores and show up on your face, hair, and nails. Wrinkles, blotchy patches, acne, and blemishes appear. Your complexion may start to look sallow, grayish, or discolored. There are more bad hair days than you care to mention. And your fingernails can turn yellow, split easily, or develop white spots, which are major alert signals that vital nutrients are lacking. Your body has become deficient in major nutrients like vitamin A, the wrinkle fighter; B complex, the stress-and-strain buffer; C, the collagen builder; E, the rejuvenator; and the beautifying minerals zinc, manganese, and magnesium, which are also needed for eliminating environmental toxins in the liver's detoxification pathways. The bottom-line result is that your system is actually aging prematurely!

Where do these toxins come from? Literally everywhere, from the environmental poisons in our air and water to the high-sugar, preserved, and processed fast foods in our diets. The landmark 1989 Kellogg Report stated, "There are over 1,000 newly synthesized compounds introduced each year, which amounts to three new chemicals a day." But many of these chemicals, we are now learning, are not just ordinary chemicals. They are petrochemicals found in pesticides, plastics, household cleaners, automobile exhaust, and even makeup, hair dyes, and everyday beauty products like fingernail polish and polish remover. Petrochemicals are known as xenobiotics or xenoestrogens, which function as hormone disrupters. And xenoestrogens include such exotic substances as bisphenol-A, found in the lining of the inside of tin cans; phthalates, contained in the plastic wrappings that leach into foods; and pesticides.

Dramatically brought to the public's attention by leading environmental scientist Theo Colburn, xenoestrogens are widely recognized as being highly potent, fat soluble, nonbiodegradable, and extremely toxic even in the smallest of doses. They are characterized as hormone disrupters because these petrochemicals have a molecular structure similar to estrogens and so interfere with the body's natural receptor sites.

The female body can play host to many toxins that can clog up the detoxification pathways and, consequently, make you look puffy and bloated. But xenoestrogens can potentially affect more than your beauty. They also trick your body into a condition known as estrogen excess or estrogen dominance. Thrown into hormone havoc, your system is now prey to diseases such as arthritis, lupus, MS, and even breast cancer. In fact, women are clearly on the front lines of the xenobiotic battle. According to John J. Condemi, M.D., clinical professor of medicine at the University of Rochester School of Medicine and Dentistry in New York, "Estrogen somehow allows the autoimmune illness to occur more readily." Health researcher Judi Vance states that the ratio of women who suffer from rheumatoid arthritis compared to men is three to one; out of the one-half to one million cases of lupus, a staggering 90 percent are female; and 230,000 of the 250–350,000 multiple sclerosis sufferers are women.

Estrogen dominance could be the underlying cause for a wide variety of symptoms you may be experiencing, from headaches and fatigue to bloating, gas, flulike symptoms, and even allergic reactions such as hives, stuffy or running noses, sneezing, and coughing. Not to mention the toxic clues on your skin, hair, and nails: rashes, acne, eczema, psoriasis, hives, or petachiae (red spots), dark circles, dry hair, yellowish nails, and so forth. When these red flags appear, covering them up with concealers or other makeup won't make them go away. Your body is sending a clear message: it's time to detoxify your system.

But in order for the liver to function properly and detoxify the system effectively, it needs support from many of the beautifying nutrients I mentioned earlier to help transform and eliminate toxins through the liver's detoxification pathways. Other special detox dietary factors are needed, such as protein to help the liver produce enzymes essential to break down hormones; cleansing high-fiber vegetables and fruits to keep the detox process moving; and beautifying, therapeutic oils to attract oil-soluble poisons lodged in fatty tissues. This is why chapters 3 to 7 provide seasonal detox principles and a revolutionary, easy-to-follow plan called the Living Beauty Detox Diet to help you prevent, control, and repair the damage toxins have caused while working to restore balance in your body. You'll learn how to nourish key organs for each season: the liver in spring; the heart and small intestines in summer; the lungs and large intestines in autumn; and the kidneys and adrenals in winter. This extremely beneficial and timely approach will help your body look and feel its best in every season, throughout every age and stage of your life.

Mental, Emotional, Spiritual Blocks: Healing Your Body, Mind, and Spirit

Many of my clients report that once their physical bodies have been cleansed of waste materials, they are ready to cleanse and rejuvenate other areas of their lives. After a seasonal cleanse of the physical body, it seems like an appropriate time for a rebirth of your emotional and psychological being. It's time to take your beauty quest to deeper levels so you can uncover your entire beauty potential. Rodin, the famous French artist and sculptor, once said, "Beauty is but the spirit breaking through the flesh." And that's the final step to achieving living beauty. You must uncover or rediscover that unique, sparkling essence deep inside you and allow it to manifest for the entire world to see.

Unlocking your individual beauty means getting in touch with and accepting who you really are, not who the images of TV ads, your friends, or relatives say you should be. But like an archaeologist on a wondrous dig, you cannot find that hidden treasure (the true beauty in you waiting to be discovered) without carefully sweeping away the dust and debris that's been covering it up all these years. You need to remove the mental, emotional, and spiritual blocks that have been hindering your personal growth because, like the toxins in your physical body, they, too, can be reflected on your face in the form of frozen facial expressions of grief, depression, and sadness.

Remember Oscar Wilde's *The Picture of Dorian Gray*? The story was about a young, handsome man who sold his soul to remain young and attractive forever. A painted portrait of his likeness bore the ugliness of his evil deeds so his physical characteristics would remain unchanged. But when the painting was destroyed, his insidious ways seeped through and became visible on his body. Finally his true essence—complete with vengeful attitudes and corruption—was exposed. It may be fiction, but the truth is your body really does have a knack of responding to thoughts and emotions. When you're feeling sad, your face looks somber. If you're happy, your eyes sparkle.

Here's the good news: you can create radiant inner and outer health by learning how to work through mental, emotional, and physical blocks. In chapter 9, I'll share with you some tried-and-true techniques and insights that have helped me on my own quest for beauty and discovery of self. As you tap into these, you also can begin to gain a deeper sense of how precious and unique you are while learning to accept and love yourself.

Living Beauty

Get ready, because living beauty—*your* beauty—is just steps away. As you journey through the next ten chapters of this book, you'll:

- learn the essential principles of detoxification so you create a powerhouse beauty foundation

- decipher your body's beauty and health SOS signals and be able to tell which detox type you are

- cleanse with seasonal detox and maintenance programs, vital for establishing a healthy inside and a beautiful outside

- rebuild and regenerate with a full spectrum of beauty nutrients

- protect your beauty by learning how to minimize the level of toxins in your physical environment

- unlock suppressed emotions so you can learn to love yourself and nurture your soul throughout your life

- zero in on your specific beauty needs for your specific age and stage of life

Remember, no matter what age or stage of life you are in, it's never too late to discover and honor your remarkable, unique self.

2

The Road to Ruin
Is Paved with
Good Intentions

Vitality and beauty are gifts of nature for
those who live according to its laws.
LEONARDO DA VINCI

Take a look in the mirror. What do you see? Red spots, dark circles, flaking skin, sallow complexion, brittle or splitting nails, thinning or strawlike hair, or maybe some other "gosh, this really makes me look yucky" beauty problem? Don't despair. Your skin (and that includes its extension, your nails and hair) acts as a window to your health and is letting you know that something could be out of balance in your body. You're not alone. Like most women, you probably have been trying hard to do all the "right" things—avoid fats at all costs, curb those carbs, take the Pill, wear sunscreen, and even supplement with calcium. But what you may not realize is that all those good intentions could be causing many of the health and hormonal problems now showing up on your skin, hair, and nails.

Good Intention #1: Fat-Free Diets

The women who have suffered the most with the fat-free mentality are those who were born in the 1970s and have come of age in the 1990s. They strongly resist consuming fat despite the updated diet trends focusing on higher protein and lower carbohydrates. When many of my own clients in their teens and twenties first came to see me, they so badly wanted to avoid gaining weight that they were subsisting on lettuce, fat-free yogurt, bagels, diet sodas, no-fat salad dressings, low-fat or no-fat cookies, white instant rice, and fat-free potato chips. Their initial diet histories revealed they were missing not only beauty and hormone-balancing oils, but also the fat-soluble antioxidants like vitamins A and E, which are essential for clear skin, resilient nails, lovely hair, and strong immunity. Moreover, because of their diet of refined white flour, these wayward beauty seekers were sorely lacking critical nutrients for detoxification, like the B vitamins, magnesium, and zinc, which help to promote hormonal balance by breaking down estrogen in the liver. Consequently, many of them were experiencing PMS symptoms, such as tender breasts, sugar cravings, and mood swings as well as fatigue, irritability, bloating, and depression.

Are you a fat-phobic female searching for beauty and "nutrition" in all the wrong places? Out of pure habit, your breakfast might consist of a bagel grabbed at a local convenience store on the way to school or a low-fat muffin with a smear of no-fat cream cheese you bought off the deli cart at work. Lunch is pasta covered in tomato sauce with a salad on the side drenched in fat-free dressing. And when dinner rolls around, it usually consists of a quick stir-fry with rice, vegetables, and a couple ounces of chicken breasts sautéed in fat-free chicken broth. If this sounds even remotely familiar, listen up: your attempt to look and feel good is in reality undermining your physical beauty, inner vitality, and overall health.

Instead, try this surefire formula for beauty and well-being:

beautifying oils + tissue-building proteins + energizing carbohydrates = healthful beauty

Beauty-enhancing oils (essential fatty acids), from both the omega-3 and omega-6 fatty acid families, are absolutely critical to your looks.

They give you dewy skin, shining hair, and healthy-looking nails by aiding in the absorption of beautifying vitamins A, D, E, and K, by producing hormones, and by helping to transport oxygen throughout your body. And they are also the gatekeepers of your appearance by helping to ward off eczema, dandruff, psoriasis, dryness, and hair loss. Primo beauty makers, these essential oils help keep cell membranes lubricated and ensure that they function properly to battle viruses and bacteria. They also help keep your body's detoxification process humming along by grabbing oil-soluble poisons stored in your fatty tissues and transporting them out for elimination. Proving their value on every level, these key power players protect your body against aging prematurely, against osteoporosis, arthritis, heart disease, cancer, allergies, and asthma.

The omega-3 fatty acids—flaxseeds, flaxseed oil, hempseed oil, pumpkin seeds, walnuts, and dark leafy greens top the list—even help to slow down the progress of yeast overgrowth in the body, which has been linked to many digestive and reproductive symptoms as well as recurrent bladder infections and skin conditions such as acne and itchy, scaly rashes. The phytohormone fiber called lignans in flax can normalize estrogen metabolism, helping to decrease PMS symptoms and the risk of breast cancer. In fact, research done by noted biochemist Jeffrey Bland, Ph.D., with omega-3 fatty acids (from flaxseed and fish oils) demonstrated a "marked impact upon the development of breast cancer" (*Nutrition Research,* vol. 9, 1989, pp. 283–93). For older women, the lignans in flaxseed with their hormone-balancing activity reduce postmenopausal hot flashes and vaginal dryness and might also help prevent osteoporosis. The omega-6 fatty acids, found in unrefined and unprocessed vegetable oils, can convert into GLA (gamma linolenic acid), which researchers have found helps to produce healthy hair, skin, and nails. GLA has also been found to stimulate brown fat metabolism, a special fat-burning tissue that dissipates excess calories for heat rather than depositing them for storage as fat. And that translates into your losing weight!

If you're staying away from protein foods, like eggs and red meat, because of the misguided notion that protein is a major fat source, you're also omitting some vital beautifying nutrients and weakening your detoxification process, not to mention playing Russian roulette with your hair, skin, and nails. Protein is important for so many reasons, like maintaining steady blood sugar and energy levels and stimulating the production of glucagon, a hormone that promotes the burning of fat for energy. Protein is also involved with tissue growth and repair; improving muscular tone; boosting metabolism by stimulating thyroid and adrenal function; and maintaining healthy hair, nails, and skin. In fact, your hair, skin, and nails are 98 percent protein. So it's no wonder that eating too little protein can cause limp hair, dull nails, droopy skin, wrinkles, soft muscle tone, and sagging breasts! Of course, the protein you consume must be healthy—organic meat, poultry, and eggs, which are not pumped up with hormones or injected with large doses of antibiotics to fight infections.

Protein plays a crucial role in detoxification by helping to carry toxins and heavy metals out of the body. And that includes excess copper, which is so prevalent these days because of copper water pipes, copper cookware, the copper IUD, the Pill, multivitamins, vegetarian diets, and copper-rich chocolate, tea, and soy. A copper overload in the system creates a zinc deficiency, because copper and zinc are antagonistic to one another. Zinc, the beautifying mineral, is also vital for strengthening hair and nails, producing clear, unblemished skin, helping bruises and wounds heal easily, and maintaining regularity in menses. It's especially critical to perimenopausal women since zinc aids with the absorption of bone-building vitamin D and helps in the bone-building formation of osteoblast cells. So when your system has a copper-induced zinc deficiency, not only is your immunity impaired, but your beauty and health suffer as well.

Elevated copper levels deplete vitamin C and the bioflavonoids, resulting in weakened collagen and elastin formation (needed for taut, young-looking skin). Because copper helps to form pigment in the skin, having too much copper in your system can lead to patches of skin with darkened pigmentation. Other beauty symptoms of copper overload and zinc deficiency can include rosacea, redness, broken capillaries, skin rashes, and white spots on the fingernails. Furthermore, when excess copper is retained in the tissues, it becomes bio-unavailable and the ability of the liver to eliminate toxins is diminished. Copper is needed in bio-available form to activate the liver's detox enzymes. A sluggish liver, in turn, is unable to break down hormones.

Good Intention #2: Carbohydrate-Free Diets

Although many of us have adopted the lower-carbohydrate, higher-protein, and higher-fat eating plans like Beyond Pritikin, The Zone, or The Atkins Diet, many women are still missing the boat on balanced nutrition and, consequently, a more balanced beauty. These women, who are typically about thirty-five years and older, have concocted their own version of the currently chic low-carbohydrate diets by flat-out eating *no* carbohydrates at all. This reminds me of the fat-free mentality of the early 1980s and '90s (as previously discussed), when many of us eliminated all fats, even the essential ones so critical to health and beauty. We're once again throwing out the baby with the bathwater on this carbohydrate issue. Cutting out all carbs, including antioxidant-rich, colorful vegetables and fruits, means losing out on rejuvenating chlorophyll, enzymes, vitamins, minerals, and cleansing fiber. Potent compounds, like the powerful phytonutrients listed below, aid in strengthening your cells and combating free radicals, which cause premature aging, robbing you of your beauty and vitality. As a matter of fact, these incredible phytonutrients also hold a star role in the fight against cancer—a major fear of women everywhere—by diffusing tumor growth in a number of ways:

- by putting the kick back in the immune system and helping to keep it in tip-top working order

- by lessening the blow from radiation, hormones, and other pollutants

- by using their estrogenlike structure to trick cancerous cells to absorb them

- by nullifying insidious enzymes produced by cancer cells to trap healthy cells

- by throwing up roadblocks so cancer cells can't stick to the surface of healthy cells

- by stopping free radicals dead in their tracks so they can't stimulate cancerous growth

What about you: Are you getting your daily dose of these antiaging phytonutrients? Here's a helpful list of foods rich in these beauty- and health-protecting nutrients:

Phytonutrient	Where Found
carotenoids	broccoli, cantaloupe, carrots, papaya, spinach, yellow squash, sweet potatoes
catechins	green and black teas
flavonoids	cabbage, carrots, citrus fruits, cucumbers, tomatoes, yams, soy foods and beverages
indoles	broccoli, brussels sprouts, cabbage, cauliflower, kale, kohlrabi, mustard greens
isoflavones	beans, peas, lentils
isothiocyanates	greens, rutabagas, turnips
lignans	nuts and seeds
limonoids	citrus fruits
lutein	spinach
monoterpenos	broccoli, cabbage, carrots, citrus fruits, yams, parsley, peppers, tomatoes, eggplant
omega-3 fatty acids	flaxseed and walnuts
organosulfur	garlic, leeks, onions, shallots
protease inhibitors	soy foods and beverages
sterole	cucumbers, eggplant, peppers, soy foods and beverages, whole grains, cereals
triterpenes	licorice root

Many of the same women who have gone on a carbohydrate-free craze are also not buying organic protein, since they believe that all protein is created equal. But the truth is, eating protein that is not organic will give you a lot more than you bargained for—like a huge dose of secondhand hormones, which will, in time, end up in the fatty tissues of the body, such as the breasts, and contribute to more estrogen excess in the body. Nonorganic meat, eggs, and poultry come from animals that have been fattened up with hormones and given heavy doses of antibiotics to ward off infections. To make the estrogen excess even worse, these animals usually have been fed grains and feed that were sprayed with pesticides and herbicides containing xenohormones, which they also pass along to us. So eating nonorganic animal foods and fats instead of healthy, therapeutic oils like flaxseed, evening primrose oil, and olive oil only adds fuel to the fire. Since xenohormones tend to settle in fat deposits—in both humans and animals—eating animal fats as part of the highprotein, lower-carbohydrate diet plans places you at further risk for another dose of these toxic estrogen mimics and their topsy-turvy, beauty-disrupting hormonal side effects.

Good Intention #3: Sunscreen

I'm sure you're well aware that overexposure to the sun creates wrinkles and brown spots, damages collagen, and reduces skin elasticity. You've heard for some time now that you should never go outdoors without sunscreen protection. So either you are barricading yourself indoors most of the time or daring to venture outdoors only after slapping on the highest level of sunscreen on the market. (Hopefully, you're choosing products that protect you from both the sun's ultraviolet rays, those short UVB rays, which cause sunburn and sun damage, as well as the far more penetrating UVA rays, the longer rays that don't cause sunburn but have been linked to skin cancer.) Ironically, your lack of sun exposure and regular use of sunscreens can actually be causing you a number of overlooked health problems and even helping to promote the skin cancer you're trying to avoid.

A certain amount of natural sunlight is essential for survival, helping to increase metabolism, regulate hormones and biorhythms, and balance moods. If you get too little sunlight, you could develop a vitamin D deficiency. Known appropriately enough as the sunshine vitamin, vitamin D helps guard against melanoma and other cancers. Vitamin D is also essential for calcium absorption and bone mineralization, so if you have too little, you will have soft bones. Consequently, a vitamin D deficiency can lead to osteoporosis and bone fractures. At least 75 percent of your body's vitamin D supply is made when a type of cholesterol in the skin is exposed to ultraviolet light. According to research published in the *Journal of Clinical Endocrinology and Metabolism* in 1987 and the *Archives of Dermatology* in 1988, sunscreens absorb the ultraviolet rays needed for your body to synthesize vitamin D, and constant sunscreen use has been found to decrease levels of vitamin D in the blood.

Alarmingly, several recent studies suggest that low levels of vitamin D in the blood increase the risk of colon cancer, breast cancer, and ovarian cancer. And another study, after discovering that the incidence of colon cancer was almost three times higher in New York than in New Mexico, concluded that a vitamin D deficiency was the likely cause since there's less exposure to sunshine in northern states. Similarly, other studies have suggested that the higher rates of both breast and ovarian cancers in the northern areas of the country are also linked to a vitamin D deficiency resulting from the lack of sunshine.

Although all the effects of a vitamin D deficiency are unknown, it's safe to say that receiving adequate D is important for promoting optimal health. Bear in mind that most of the world's population relies on natural, unprotected exposure to sunlight to maintain adequate vitamin D nutrition. Not a lot of sunshine is necessary for vitamin D synthesis. Estimates on the amount of sun exposure time needed vary from fifteen minutes to one hour daily.

Good Intention #4: Birth Control Pills

Taking a proactive approach to contraception is smart. But are popular methods doing more harm than good by destroying your looks and health? Sometimes taking the Pill can cause already excessive estrogen levels to soar, making skin dark with blotchy brown patches called melasma. While today's pills, like Alesse and LoEstrin (1/20), contain considerably less estrogen (20 mcg. of estrogen) than the older versions

(80 mcg. of estrogen), keep in mind that you are still ingesting estrogen. And your body is already fighting excess estrogens from the environment (in the form of the plastics, pesticides, and hormone-packed food), which are disrupting your delicate hormonal balance. Adding more estrogen to the mix only compounds the problem. A Harvard study of more than 65,000 nurses that was published in the prestigious *New England Journal of Medicine* (June 15, 1995) reported that in women sixty to sixty-five who were on estrogen replacement for five years or longer there was a 71 percent higher risk of breast cancer. And because copper retention has been associated with estrogen supplementation, copper-overload symptoms can manifest in hair loss and skin problems plus a variety of troubling symptoms like fatigue, anxiety, panic attacks, and insomnia. As mentioned earlier, a copper excess means a deficiency in the beauty fortifier, zinc. Interestingly, zinc levels have a dramatic connection to eating disorders, since zinc is a necessary nutrient for the appetite control center of the brain. As a matter of fact, leading researchers clinically linked anorexia with zinc deficiencies as far back as 1979. In that year, Dr. R. Bakan said in "The Role of Zinc in Anorexia Nervosa: Etiology and Treatment," in *Medical Hypotheses*, that females between the ages of twelve and twenty-five are most at risk not only for anorexia but also for chronic zinc deficiencies.

The Pill can also cause a number of nutrient deficiencies that result in a host of beauty and hormonal problems. Among them are a deficiency in B_6, causing dandruff, hair loss, thinning hair, dermatitis and stretch marks, PMS, changes in the menstrual cycle, and a decrease in estrogen-balancing progesterone; a deficiency in B_{12}, resulting in that rundown, haggard look and anemia; low levels of biotin, resulting in hair loss, dry hair, eczema, brittle nails, and fatigue; in folic acid, resulting in a sallow complexion, premature graying, poor skin color, and a form of anemia; in vitamin C, affecting collagen production, wrinkle formation, bruising, and capillary strength; in vitamin E, causing sagging facial muscles, weaknesses in connective tissue, varicose veins, and fluctuating estrogen levels that yield PMS and perimenopausal symptoms; in zinc, resulting in acne, blemishes, easy bruising, and a decrease in estrogen-balancing progesterone.

Good Intention #5: Calcium Craze

No doubt you've read about how important calcium is for beautiful teeth and bones. Like many women, in addition to eating calcium-rich dairy foods, you may also be popping calcium-fortified antacids, drinking calcium-fortified juices, and eating calcium-fortified dairy products. But wait! A new study reveals, like others before it, that too much calcium may actually weaken strong bones. A two-year study of approximately 9,000 women who were sixty-five years of age or older, published in the *American Journal of Epidemiology* (vol. 145, 1997), showed no significant relationship between taking calcium and "the risk of any of the fractures studied." Calcium supplementation as well as supplementation with Tums actually increased the risk of hip fracture. For many of my readers of *Super Nutrition for Menopause* (Avery, 1998) and *Before the Change* (HarperSanFrancisco, 1998), this should come as no surprise. I have always maintained that it is not calcium but *magnesium* that is the real mineral catalyst in the absorption and use of bone-building elements.

Others agree. Researcher and gynecologist Dr. Guy Abraham published a widely quoted study in the *Journal of Reproductive Medicine* (vol. 35, May 1990) entitled "A Total Dietary Program Emphasizing Magnesium Instead of Calcium: Effect on the Mineral Density of Calcaneous Bone in Postmenopausal Women on Hormonal Therapy." His study demonstrated an amazing 11 percent bone density increase in just one year after more magnesium than calcium was ingested from food and supplemental sources. The dose was 600–1,000 mg. of magnesium plus 500 mg. of calcium for one year. In addition, Israeli research published in the *Medical Tribune* (July 22, 1993) reported a study demonstrating an increase in bone density of 8 percent when magnesium was singly used (without any calcium at all) in supplements ranging from 250 mg. to 750 mg.

According to nutrition expert Nan Kathryn Fuchs, Ph.D., who has worked clinically with Dr. Abraham, "Excessive calcium prevents the absorption of magnesium. Taking more calcium without adequate magnesium—and what is adequate for one woman may be insufficient for another—may either create calcium malabsorption or a magnesium deficiency." Unabsorbed calcium can wind up in the joints as arthritis or in the arteries where it can initiate atherosclerosis. As Fuchs so aptly observes, heart disease is the number one killer of postmenopausal women—the very age group that is overloading on calcium because of the misguided notion that more is better when it comes to building strong bones.

Besides warding off both heart disease and osteoporosis, magnesium, the unsung female guardian angel, aids in the absorption of B vitamins and helps to break down estrogen in the liver, thus aiding in PMS, peri-menopausal, and menopausal discomforts ranging from mood swings to anxiety to insomnia.

Good Intention #6: Trying to Stay Beautiful and Healthy amidst Modern-Day Hazards

Despite the fact that the world is forging ahead with the latest and great-est technology, your fingertips are cracking, your nails are breaking too easily, and your skin is often covered with rashes, bumps, blackheads, and pimples. Why? It's simple. You're living in a chemical world.

Since World War II, a whole new breed of toxins has come into use, known as xenoestrogens, which in the body mimic estrogen. These poiso-nous infiltrators are spearheading a continual assault on your beauty and health in the form of pesticides, plastics, solvents, automobile exhaust, industrial chemicals, food additives, and environmental pollutants. To give you an idea of what your body is up against, take a look at these U.S. statistics from 1995 to 1996. Every year:

- 2.4 billion pounds of industrial chemicals pollute our air

- 240 million tons of hazardous waste congest landfills

- 20–30 tons of waste are produced from just one nuclear reactor

These toxic substances enter your body in a number of ways, via the skin, food, or nostrils, and are contributing to a relatively new condition within the past fifty years known as estrogen dominance. Estrogen in properly balanced amounts is a skin firmer and hydrator, an antidepressant, and a mood and memory enhancer; however, an excess is an entirely different matter. Symptoms of estrogen dominance look strikingly like PMS, perimenopausal, and menopausal symptoms. The picture is further compounded by a lack of the calming hormone known as progesterone—meaning "for gestation"—which counters excess estrogen's negative and often irritating, excitable effects. Touted as the "feel-good hormone," progesterone is up to twenty times more concentrated in the brain than in the bloodstream.

Progesterone is widely recognized today thanks to the pioneering research of Dr. Raymond Peat and Dr. John Lee. Having a progesterone deficiency is epidemic among women from eighteen to eighty. Many women's bodies simply aren't producing enough because they lack the nutrient precursors zinc and vitamin B_6, because they are not ovulating regularly and so there is no corpus luteum to create progesterone, and because their bodies are converting progesterone into other chemicals on account of excessive stress. Progesterone can negate the effects of excess estrogen by lubricating your skin, acting as a natural diuretic, transforming fat into energy, helping to stabilize blood-sugar levels, aiding in thyroid and hormone functions, and preventing cysts and cancerous cells to grow in your breasts. Between natural hormonal fluctuations and the environmental xenohormones assaulting your body, a number of beauty and health issues can manifest, from whiskers on the chin to thinning hair and breaking capillaries to yeast infections, irritability, irregular periods, aging or dry skin, acne, liver or age spots, weight gain, and mood fluctuations.

Good Intentions Infinitum

And if all that wasn't enough, a whole other slew of "good" things you may be using every day not only get in the way of radiant beauty and vibrant health but also lead to disease. A shocking report published in the prestigious British medical journal *The Lancet* back in 1979 linked talcum powder—you know, the soft, clean-smelling stuff you've been sprinkling all over your body since you were so high—to ovarian cancer. Over ten years later, in 1992, the National Cancer Institute conducted an investigation on permanent hair dyes, which showed that women who use them have a 50 percent higher risk of non-Hodgkin's lymphoma (a relatively rare cancer), the same cancer that took the life of former first lady Jacqueline Kennedy. The coal tar colors found in black, brown, and red dyes were implicated, whereas lighter colors or semipermanent dyes were not. And these same coal tar colors are also found in certain foundations, blushers, and lipstick today.

Not only are cosmetics creating trouble, but many of the medications you use daily can contribute to the war against your health as well. Living in a fast-paced world, you've come to expect fast answers and fast relief. So you may not even think twice about running down to your local drugstore to grab aspirin or ibuprofen for a quick fix for those coldlike symptoms. But when these over-the-counter products are used to squelch pain or fever during a cold, they've been shown to suppress immune response, boost viral action, and make a runny nose worse. In fact, antihistamines along with other similar medications cause tear ducts and salivary glands to dry up. Antibiotics aren't any better. Although they hold an important role in our lives, antibiotics tend to disrupt the natural balance of the gastrointestinal tract by destroying both the beneficial and harmful bacteria. And that opens up the door for parasitic invasion and allows yeast in the gut to grow unchecked. Did you know that just one yeast cell can produce over 70 toxic substances that will eventually compromise the immune system, glands, and other major organs such as the kidneys, bladder, and liver?

Even our good intentions with clean and pure water are causing a health backlash, as you will read about later. The chlorine used to disinfect municipal water supplies is a xenoestrogen that contributes to a hormonal imbalance in your system. Here's a startling fact: your body absorbs more chlorine in a short ten-minute shower than it would if you drank eight glasses of the same water!

U-Turn

As you can see, many well-intended but misguided eating habits and lifestyle practices have created a whole new group of beauty and health issues that have become more problematic than the original concern. They can affect you throughout your entire life cycle. Moreover, as you will learn in the following chapters, the nutritional deficiencies resulting from your good intentions (lack of the right fats, organic proteins, phytonutrient-rich carbohydrates, and minerals like zinc and magnesium) have inhibited the body's ability to detoxify all the poisons polluting your system.

That's why it is high time to turn beauty inside out by ridding the tissues of stored toxins, following the body's natural detoxification cycle each season. Each of the specially designed detox plans—for spring, summer, autumn, and winter—incorporates seasonally available vegetables and fruits high in cleansing enzymes and purifying fiber as well as tissue-strengthening proteins and beautifying oils for the most scientifically sound cleansing. Undergoing a seasonal cleansing four times a year will improve your hair, skin, and nails immeasurably; it will energize you and increase mental clarity; it will help to balance PMS, perimenopausal, and menopausal discomforts; and it will make those unwanted pounds disappear and reduce cellulite.

As you embark on your journey for more healthful beauty, this book will show you how to cleanse your body throughout the year with the seasonal Living Beauty Detox Diet plans. It will provide you with follow-up maintenance diet tips, then present the Living Beauty Alphabet of Vitamins and Minerals, which will guarantee that you're looking your absolute, all-time best after you've flushed away the toxins. Now, what could be better?

3

Seasonal Beauty:

Internal Cleansing and Support for Spring, Summer, Fall, Winter

*Whoever wishes to investigate medicine should
proceed thus: In the first place consider the seasons
of the year and what effect each produces.*
HIPPOCRATES

In this chapter you'll learn a revolutionary approach to help you look and feel renewed by eating to detoxify your system. No matter when you're reading this book—spring, summer, autumn, winter—you can start this program at any point. Just read the general overview and diet components, then follow the suggestions listed for the season you're in. If it's summer, start with the summer plan; in winter, begin with the winter plan. Before long, you'll have more energy, better elimination, and the radiant skin you long for.

Believe me, it works. As a firm believer that detoxification is the missing link to health and vitality, I've shown hundreds of women how the Living Beauty Detox Program works beauty miracles. It is undoubtedly the reason that I can keep up with a demanding lifestyle and still maintain well-being, and you can, too. With the specially designed cleansing plans that allow you to both cleanse your system and support your energy throughout the day, you'll learn how to eat your way through detoxification while targeting specific organs of your body according to the various seasons.

The Living Beauty Detox Diet

My seasonal detox method—your personal guide to discovering beauty from the inside out—targets major detoxification pathways and is based on the Traditional Chinese Medicine approach to health throughout the year. The Chinese understood that the Earth has its seasonal periods when certain organs are more vulnerable and need special care. So in the Living Beauty Detox Diet, you'll detoxify, rebuild, and nurture the organs of your body that the Chinese for centuries have believed correlate with a particular time of year. You'll focus on your liver and gall bladder in the spring; heart and small intestine in the summer; lungs and large intestine in the autumn; then kidneys and adrenals in the winter.

But Earth's cycles are more than a wise guideline for caring for vital organs and clearing your detoxification pathways. The Earth's seasons affect you on emotional and hormonal levels as well. You've probably already known how dampness, rain, and cold, harsh winters can chill your bones and aggravate certain health conditions. But the dwindling sunlight of autumn and winter can also take its toll on your health and emotions.

The New Way to Detoxify: No More Fasting

In this revolutionary program, you'll notice an extremely important difference from other detox plans—no fasting! You will, as I mentioned above, be eating your way through the detoxification process. You may have heard that fasting, which is the absence of food and drink except for water, is one of the fastest ways to stimulate the body to release toxins, since the stress of digestion is removed. However, groundbreaking research that was published in *Alternative Therapies in Health and Medicine* in 1995 and conducted by Jeffrey Bland, Ph.D., director of the

HealthComm Clinical Research Center in Gig Harbor, Washington, has clearly demonstrated that the body's built-in detoxification pathways require heavy nutritional support every step of the way. Therefore, fasting to detoxify the body may actually hinder the process.

Because fasting accelerates the burning of fatty tissue where many toxins are stored, an overload of toxic compounds can be dumped into the bloodstream and impair the liver's detoxification pathways, resulting in toxic metabolites, much more harmful than the original substances. So fasting actually retards the liver's ability to detoxify your system. Earlier research reported by Dr. Bland in the *Journal of Applied Nutrition* (vols. 3–4, Feb. 15, 1992) states that in animal studies, the enzyme systems in the liver significantly decreased their output within thirty-six hours after fasting. Simply put, when detox enzymes are not working, hormones like estrogen cannot be broken down. And for us females, this leads to estrogen dominance, with symptoms that mimic PMS, perimenopause, and menopause: crankiness, bloating, and other not-so-charming side effects hardly conducive to beauty!

Fasting also drains the body of vital antioxidants like glutathione needed to support the detox process. Glutathione is the predominant player against toxic oxygen radicals. It's typically found in high levels in the liver and other organs in the detox system. When the liver is exposed to an increased amount of poisons, more glutathione is in demand to properly break the toxins down. Glutathione has also earned the nickname of "the toxic waste neutralizer of the body" or "nature's antiaging agent" because this powerful nutrient stands on the front lines defending your body against disease, aging, cancer, and toxins.

It does this by helping to fight against both free radicals and oxygen radicals and by regulating the functions of other antioxidants, such as vitamins A, C, and E. Did you know that the most widely accepted theory of aging today is that it is caused by free radicals? They damage our cells and tissues by weakening and altering cell membranes, which allow bacteria and viruses to enter the body. They also destroy genetic coding, resulting in cellular chaos and deterioration of all tissues and organs, including the brain. So it is imperative that we don't deplete this valuable antioxidant, glutathione, by restricting food or fasting. If we do, dangerous secondary metabolites will roam freely and work their damage on the liver and other organs. These threatening metabolites can produce severe consequences to the immune, nervous, and endocrine systems.

Plain and simple, juice fasting is not only antiquated, it can be downright dangerous. Although juice provides readily absorbed vitamins, minerals, and enzymes—some of which, like vitamins A, C, and B complex, are necessary cofactors in the detox process—juices do not contain protein. And lack of protein not only opens the door to an increase in production of secondary toxins by the liver but can also lead to muscle tissue catabolism, which means our bodies actually start to break down muscle tissue to get energy.

Eat Your Way to Beauty

So what exactly does the Living Beauty Detox Diet include? Everything you'll need to support your body nutritionally and protect it against potential damage from free radicals and other toxins produced during the two phases of the detoxification process. The liver is the Grand Central Station, so to speak, of your body's functions, especially for both phases of the detoxification processes. As the largest internal organ, your liver sits in the right upper abdomen and helps keep the energy flow of the body in balance, regulating the blood flow, giving support to the digestive system, and even ensuring the optimal function of your menstrual cycle. In fact, every second of the day, your liver is systematically filtering and detoxifying everything that enters your body, from the food you eat down to the medications you take, protecting you from becoming poisoned. As the central clearinghouse, your liver has the sole responsibility of determining which substances are beneficial to your body and which ones need to be kicked out. And that's where the critical phases of the detox process come into play.

Your liver begins Phase 1 of the detox process by stimulating the cytochrome P-450 enzymes needed to grab hold of toxins for oxidation. This process results in another group of compounds called the intermediates. Then in Phase 2, your liver performs an enzymatic conversion transforming the intermediates from their fat-soluble form to a substance that is nontoxic, water soluble, and easily excreted. Of course, in order for both phases to function properly, your body needs the kind of nutrition vital to keeping the detox pathways running optimally, such as antioxidants, zinc, and vitamins A, C, E, B_1, and B_2 for Phase 1; and folic acid, vitamin E, selenium, manganese, glutathione, as well as the amino acids methionine, cysteine, glycine, glutamine, and taurine for Phase 2.

But all too frequently, other factors interrupt the process, such as highly refined foods, nitrates, hormones, and preservatives, along with environmental xenohormones, caffeine, alcohol, the Pill, overuse of antibiotics, over-the-counter drugs, smog, secondhand smoke, and even the metabolic residue from your food. When these elements come into play, your liver no longer performs normally, causing toxins to build up in your system, where they provoke chronic health conditions.

Your liver, as the center of action, also purifies the bloodstream; maintains blood sugar levels; produces enzymes and amino acids to metabolize carbohydrates, fats, and proteins; produces bile during the digestive process for fat metabolism, then houses the bile in the gallbladder; and helps keep your body in hormonal balance, which is particularly important in metabolizing estrogen. Your liver detoxifies the components of estrogen (estrone and estradiol) and transforms them into nontoxic substances. When a poor-functioning liver hinders this process, you could experience irregular menses, hair loss, and psoriasis and could even be at higher risk for breast cancer.

Simply put, the liver is the key to life. When your liver is sluggish, every organ in your body becomes affected by it. Your blood vessels enlarge, and blood flow becomes restricted. The congested liver starts to propel toxins into your circulatory system, producing a dull ache under your lower right rib cage (particularly after a rich meal). And with toxins running amok in your body, secondary problems are usually not far behind. The liver—which also produces enzymes and amino acids to aid in digestion—becomes overwhelmed and throws the whole body out of balance, which weakens the gastro lining and releases more toxins into the system. And as higher amounts of these poisons are released, even more make their way to your liver, which starts the insidious circle all over again.

As the seat of energy flow for the body, your liver is susceptible to stagnation problems. Unresolved or prolonged anger and depression—the emotional markers of a compromised liver—prevent the body's energy from flowing as it should. You may have a deep vertical crease between your eyebrows as a result or a dark or reddish complexion. You could also experience a myriad of secondary symptoms such as acne; itchy rashes; petachiae (red spots); splitting or breaking fingernails; hormonal imbalances, from premenstrual irritability, mood swings, and cramping to perimenopausal irritability, mental fog, anxiety, and depression to menopausal hot flashes, palpitations, and night sweats; and digestive problems. In fact, contending with years of a stress-damaged liver has also been known to bring about earlier menopausal symptoms.

Protein: The Detox Powerhouse

Critical to both phases is protein, the star performer in beauty functions. And remember, as I mentioned earlier, protein is equated with beauty since our skin, hair, and nails are 98 percent protein. This is why a protein deficiency produces hair loss, droopy facial muscles, wrinkles, and weak nails. In fact, practically every part of your body relies on protein for existence. Protein helps make the powerhouse antioxidant glutathione; assists in escorting iron and copper in the body; creates vital enzymes to zap toxins; maintains energy levels; and helps keep blood sugar in balance by supporting the adrenal glands, pancreas, and liver. And since the body can't store protein, it's essential that we get the right amount daily. Having low protein levels increases our desire for carbohydrates (like sugar), which contribute to a rise in insulin levels.

Oils: Critical for Cleansing

My unique seasonal detox program also includes specific beautifying oils for you to use in each season. These oils are essential for supple, youthful-looking skin, and luxurious hair, and they help with the vital detox process itself. No matter what the time of year, you'll have at least

one tablespoon each day of omega-3 lignan-rich flaxseed oil to help stabilize blood sugar, keep your appetite down, and combat excess estrogen in your system. Lignans are a type of fiber especially important for
fighting breast cancer. A 1997 *Lancet* study conducted by researchers
in Perth, Western Australia, found a dramatic reduction in breast cancer risk among women having a high intake of lignans, like those found
in flaxseed oil.

Besides the lignan-rich flaxseed oil, all of the therapeutic oils you'll
be taking are vital for detoxification because they also help attract the
oil-soluble poisons lodged in fatty tissues and usher them out of the system. The essential and healthy fatty acids (once known as vitamin F)
contained in the therapeutic oils are an integral part of the program
because they produce hormones; facilitate oxygen transportation; help
absorb fat-soluble vitamins A, D, E, and K; and are essential for great-
looking skin and hair.

Vegetables: Cornerstone of Necessary Nutrients

Eating the right kinds and amounts of vegetables and fruits is not only
beneficial for your health and beauty; it is also absolutely crucial for
the detoxification process. So as you eat your way to health, you can
choose from a colorful array of fruits and vegetables that are low on the
glycemic index. Many, like yellow squash, greens, and tomatoes, contain phytonutrients (for example, carotenoids and flavonoids essential
in fortifying cell membranes to renew and regenerate the integrity of
your skin). Plus, fruits and vegetables are natural resources for other
health-promoting antioxidants like vitamins C and E as well as zinc,
selenium, and, to a lesser degree, glutathione.

But remember, your goal is to flush toxins from your body to restore
hormonal harmony, which produces the beautifying effects of silkier hair,
polished skin, a slimmed-down waist, and no more bloating. This is why
the Living Beauty Detox Diet emphasizes organic or purified foods.
Organic fruits and vegetables (unlike conventionally grown produce) is
pesticide free and is grown in healthy soil that hasn't been tainted by
chemical fertilizers or additives. Nonorganic produce is grown in mineral-
depleted soils and is sprayed with pesticides, herbicides, and fungicides,

many of which are considered xenohormonic. You've already read how these estrogen mimics can create a playground for hormones that ends up in utter mayhem, reducing the liver's ability to eliminate and function optimally.

If you aren't able to purchase organic fruits and vegetables, please be sure to wash your produce in a hydrogen-peroxide bath to remove chemicals. This method offers an added bonus because it also helps keep your food fresher longer. Simply get a dishpan or similar container and mix:

¼ cup of 3 percent hydrogen peroxide (found at the grocery store or drugstore)

2 gallons of water (purified water is best, if you can)

Soak thin-skinned fruits (nectarines, peaches, berries) and leafy vegetables for fifteen minutes; thick-skinned fruits (oranges, lemons, apples) and thick-skinned or root vegetables for thirty minutes. After removing the fruits or vegetables, rinse and let them stand in purified water for approximately ten minutes. Then drain them and dry well.

Side note: Although I have promoted a Clorox bath for years, many people are under the assumption that Clorox is an organochlorine, a xenohormone compound found in pesticides and insecticides. The active ingredient in Clorox, however, is actually sodium hypochlorite, which breaks down into salt and water.

Herbs, Spice, and Everything Nice

Very specific healing teas, herbs, and spices are recommended in the seasonal detox programs. These herbs and spices will help to gently but effectively cleanse and nourish the detoxification pathways or organs and glands related to each season. You can make your own herbal teas or buy them locally in health food stores in ready-made tea bags. The signature teas for each season include dandelion for spring, rose hips for summer, fenugreek for autumn, and nettles for winter.

Although the other seasonal herbs are considered optional, they are highly recommended either alone or in blended formulas at breakfast and dinner for those with high levels of toxicity who will be following the program for a longer period of time. Please note that some of the more unusual herbs may not be easily available at your herb or health food store (like usnea, for example, suggested in autumn for optimum respiratory health). In this case, please refer to the Resource section for herbal mail order companies where you can purchase all the herbs that are recommended in either tincture or capsule form. Follow the instructions on the label.

Spices such as dill, oregano, garlic, cayenne, and cinnamon are included in the cleansing plans for their double whammy effect. Some (like oregano, garlic, rosemary, and thyme) are microbe-fighting spices. Others, besides providing a delightful taste, offer a rich source of trace minerals and flavonoids, mega-antioxidants critical for the detoxification process itself and enhanced immunity. Use the immune-boosting spices to add a little zing and additional healthful flavor to your menu.

Make sure your herbs (in teas, tinctures, or capsules) are certified organic and that your spices are nonirradiated. It's the oil in the spices that contains many of their health-enhancing qualities. To release the oil for its optimal health benefits, use a mortar and pestle or a small grinder.

Sugars: Beauty Busters

To decrease your toxic burden, you will not find manufactured or hydrogenated fats like margarine, shortening, or refined vegetable oils in the detox or maintenance programs. Sugar, caffeine, alcohol, and white-flour products are also banished because they sabotage the cleansing process and your overall health. While caffeine and alcohol are considered primary intestinal irritants, sugar, caffeine, alcohol, and white-flour products (like bread, rice, and pasta) all deplete B vitamins, magnesium, and zinc, which are essential cofactors for detoxification (especially in the liver's breakdown of estrogen) and for producing estrogen-balancing progesterone. Because of its sugar content, most fruit juice is omitted, and even fruits are restricted. All of these foods can throw your blood sugar off balance, which makes you feel tired. Blood sugar imbalance can also encourage candida (yeast) overgrowth in your intestines, resulting in depression and fatigue, and it drains your adrenal glands, pancreas, and thyroid gland, rendering you utterly exhausted. Plus, researchers have discovered a positive link between excessive sugar consumption and eight forms of cancer, including breast, ovary, pancreas, kidney, colon, nervous system, rectum, and prostate. The cancer risk doubled in some patients where sugar was eaten on a regular basis.

Caffeine: Adrenal Robbers

The number one caffeine product in our country—to the tune of a half-billion cups every day—is coffee. But our romantic love affair with java exposes us to hazardous health concerns. For starters, the coffee bean is brimming with rancid oils and aggravating acids. Then it's grown and processed with toxic chemicals and pesticides. And forget about switching to decaffeinated, because it's processed with health-risking agents like trichlorethylene or methylene chloride. Plus, sugar and coffee both overly activate the adrenal glands, causing them to become sluggish and eventually depleted. When that happens, your adrenals can no longer function effectively, so your blood sugar becomes unstable and you will crave the quick-fix carbohydrates that are detrimental to and actually hinder the cleansing process.

Since all of the detox plans are as hypoallergenic as possible, there are two particular food groups that you will not see appearing in the seasonal detox list: the grains (wheat, rye, oats, and barley) and dairy products. Gluten-rich grains, cereals, pasta, or bread have not only been linked to weight gain but also are associated with hidden allergic food reactions in the form of gastrointestinal problems, arthritis, headaches, and depression. Dairy products can promote sinus problems, excessive mucus, phlegm, and cellulite in many individuals. Please note, however, that nonallergic grains (cereals, pasta, and bread) and organic dairy products from organic companies are part of the more expanded maintenance program.

Before You Begin: Think Zinc

Since avoiding xenohormones, which contribute to estrogen dominance and the resulting beauty side effects of blotchy skin, thinning hair, and broken capillaries, is such an important factor in the detox programs, I'm sure you'll agree that going out of your way to locate organic oils, protein sources, and produce will be worth the beauty benefits. And to further help you combat estrogen dominance, I have purposefully included foods high in zinc (like organic red meat and organic eggs) on the detox menu plans and lots of zinc-rich pumpkin seeds on the maintenance programs. Zinc is the mineral precursor to progesterone that counters estrogen in the body. Conversely, I have limited copper-rich foods in the detox menu plan (like soy-based protein powders, tempeh, soy milk, and tofu) and in the maintenance plan (like high-copper nuts and grains). As I mentioned earlier, the mineral copper has been linked with raised estrogen levels, just as zinc has been linked to progesterone levels.

How the Detox Plan Works

You'll begin each season with a minimum three-day detox program, then you'll choose from a wide variety of seasonal foods on the delicious maintenance plan specially designed for that time of year. I emphasize the word *minimum* here because I'm sure you will want to continue the three-day program for up to two weeks and even longer once you experience the beautifying side effects of this new way of cleansing. Your skin will clear up, your hair will shine, your eyes will become brighter, your brain will be sharper, your digestion will become more efficient, and your energy will go through the roof! Not to mention that you will need less sleep and that arthritic aches and pains as well as food allergies can greatly diminish.

My specially designed minimum three-day detox is composed of organic, seasonal foods, herbal teas, and a super green food supplement, which provides key nutrients imperative for cleansing. Using this detox plan as a foundation, you will then incorporate other seasonal favorites on the delicious maintenance plan specially designed for that time of year.

Whatever the season, the following components, briefly touched upon in the previous pages, form the complete protocol of the Living Beauty Detox Diet:

- *Therapeutic Oils.* To increase your metabolic power and lubricate the system for more effective cleansing, I'll suggest taking two tablespoons of a seasonal therapeutic oil. As mentioned earlier, every season will include having at least one tablespoon of high-lignan flaxseed oil daily because the lignan fiber component is known to be helpful in detoxifying excess estrogens from the system. The high omega-3 fatty acid component of the flaxseed oil is also beneficial for overall health and well-being, not to mention the outward beauty of the skin, hair, and nails. And oil is a potent blood sugar stabilizer.

- *Lean Protein.* A component of skin, hair, nails, and muscle tissue, protein is absolutely vital to the detoxification process. You'll eat at least two servings (four ounces each—the size of the palm of your hand) per day of lean beef, veal, or lamb, skinless chicken or turkey, and all kinds of fish. Protein activates the production of the enzymes needed to break down toxins into water-soluble substances for excretion. Plus, animal proteins, unlike vegetarian sources, are high in zinc, the progesterone precursor. However, try to purchase farm-raised products as much as possible, and stay away from swordfish, which is more likely to accumulate mercury, PCBs, and other xenohormones, like dioxin. And as I stated earlier, your purpose is to rid your body of toxins, so the meat and poultry should be organically raised and hormone free. You may also eat organic eggs (one egg equals one ounce of animal protein). But since research has shown that eating egg whites by themselves increases allergic response, eat the whole egg when it is part of the menu plan. Like the oil component, all protein sources are potent blood sugar stabilizers and should curb your appetite between meals when you may be tempted to snack on carbohydrates, which will hinder the detox process. For vegetarians, high protein providers made from lactose-free whey and low carbohydrate legumes can be used as a substitute for animal protein.

- *Vegetables.* Choose organic seasonal produce that is nonstarchy and slow acting, or low glycemic, for longer-lasting energy. The high fiber content of these nonstarchy vegetables not only slows down digestion but also helps to sweep out toxins from the system like an intestinal broom. For these reasons, you may eat an unlimited amount raw or steamed. Fresh vegetables provide enzymes, vitamins, minerals, and chlorophylls for radiant good looks. You will note that no matter what the season, there are many selections of cruciferous vegetables. This is because their sulfur content helps support the detoxification process: cabbage, kale, kohlrabi, brussels sprouts, mustard greens, watercress, leeks, onion, radish, cauliflower, and horseradish.

- *Fruits.* Choose organic, mostly low-glycemic fruits of the season. Cleansing fresh fruit offers collagen-enhancing vitamin C and bioflavonoids. Fruits are also a rich source of enzyme-activating potassium, which is also a muscle strengthener. Eat two whole portions daily in the specified amounts to maintain balanced blood sugar levels. Happily, you may eat three whole portions in the summer because fruits are cooling to the body. You will be eating applesauce and various applesauce fruit blends in winter when your choice of fresh fruits is limited.

- *Living Beauty Elixir.* Twice a day—when you get up and when you go to bed—blend and drink eight ounces of unsweetened cranberry juice with two teaspoons of a green superfood mixture, rich in purifying chlorophyll and detoxifying antioxidants and nutrients (please see Resources for brand-name recommendations). Cranberry juice, a known cleanser of the urinary tract, also helps the liver to open up the detoxification pathways. Cranberry contains several digestive enzymes not found in other foods. So it's a marvelous cleanser for the lymphatic system, the most underrated system in the body. This vital system is made up of millions of tiny channels running through all parts of the body, transporting nutrients to the cells and removing wastes from the cells via the connective tissue. Dependent upon muscle contraction for its flow, the body cannot detox effectively if the lymph is not moving. Cleansing the lymphatic system, also known as the garbage collection system of the body, is the missing health and beauty link. The cranberry in the Living Beauty Elixir helps to digest stagnant lymphatic waste and helps cellulite do a disappearing act.

- *Fiber-Rich Supplement.* Along with the Beauty Elixir twice a day, include a high-fiber supplement to make sure your body is sweeping away the debris that's clogging your intestinal tract; this prevents the absorption of new toxins. Many additional cleansing herbal components that can be found in high-fiber supplements such as Irish Moss, buckthorn, butternut, and peppermint, aid the liver and intestinal tract to eliminate a wide variety of wastes and environmental toxins like heavy metals and parasites. A high-fiber supplement promotes regularity with its soluble and nonsoluble fibers like psyllium, oat bran, and powdered flaxseed. A fiber-rich supplement increases energy levels and aids in enhanced nutrient absorption without gas or bloating discomfort.

- *Purified Water.* Drinking plenty of purified, filtered water each day is vitally important for diluting and expelling toxins. But it's even more vital when you're on a detoxification program. Water ensures normal bowel and kidney functions, ridding the body of wastes as well as stored toxic fat. Adequate amounts of water will assist the kidneys in filtering their own waste products so that the liver can begin to metabolize its own waste materials without having to do the kidney's work. You must drink at least eight glasses a day to help your system stay in tip-top shape. Water has the added benefit of helping your skin stay hydrated and promotes sweating—a primary detox mechanism. Please consult the Resource section for more information on purified water.

The Living Beauty Cleansing Questionnaire

Take a moment to complete the following Living Beauty Cleansing Questionnaire. Read through the symptom list, and mark off each one according to the frequency of your experience. As you look over the list, you will notice that seemingly unrelated symptoms (like eye problems in the spring, which is the liver and gallbladder season) are listed together. This is not an oversight. According to Traditional Chinese Medicine, the acupuncture meridians connect various organs (such as the eyes and the liver) to one another. The answers you give to this questionnaire will help you accomplish two things: individualize your unique cleansing needs by understanding your personal level of toxicity, and determine which season is your dominant type. Although you may suffer from certain symptoms like dry skin and PMS throughout the year, they are generally intensified during certain seasons, which signal the time of the year to take special precautions.

Give yourself 0 points for every "rarely" answer; 3 points for every "occasionally" answer; and 5 points for every "frequently, at least once a week" answer. Then, add up your score for each section and circle your highest score. This signals your dominant season type.

	Type 1: Spring
appearance:	*sustained, reddish complexion, dark and swarthy; deep vertical crease between eyebrows*
emotional hallmarks:	*unresolved and prolonged anger and irritability*
acne, blemishes, hives, itchy rashes	__rarely __occasionally, once a month or less __frequently, at least once a week
oily facial skin and scalp	__rarely __occasionally, once a month or less __frequently, at least once a week
split or thickened nails	__rarely __occasionally, once a month or less __frequently, at least once a week
petachiae (small, red, pinheadlike blood spots that come and go on body)	__rarely __occasionally, once a month or less __frequently, at least once a week
jaundice	__rarely __occasionally, once a month or less __frequently, at least once a week
eye problems such as itchy red eyes, light sensitivity, floaters, farsightedness, myopia, sties, tearing eyes, or blurry vision	__rarely __occasionally, once a month or less __frequently, at least once a week
hemorrhoids or varicose veins	__rarely __occasionally, once a month or less __frequently, at least once a week

Continued

	Type 1: Spring, continued
hormonal imbalances, including PMS menstrual irritability, mood swings, cramping, and bloating with heavy menstrual flow and heavy clotting	__rarely __occasionally, once a month or less __frequently, at least once a week
hormonal imbalances like perimenopausal irritability, mental fog, anxiety, and depression	__rarely __occasionally, once a month or less __frequently, at least once a week
hormonal imbalances such as menopausal hot flashes, palpitations, night sweats, hair loss, and dry-eye syndrome	__rarely __occasionally, once a month or less __frequently, at least once a week
heat in the upper body (face feels hot, eyes feel hot)	__rarely __occasionally, once a month or less __frequently, at least once a week
light-colored stools	__rarely __occasionally, once a month or less __frequently, at least once a week
nauseated, especially after eating fatty foods	__rarely __occasionally, once a month or less __frequently, at least once a week
digestive problems such as gas, bloating, belching	__rarely __occasionally, once a month or less __frequently, at least once a week
rib cage sensitivity, particularly under the right ribs	__rarely __occasionally, once a month or less __frequently, at least once a week
chronic tension in neck and across shoulders	__rarely __occasionally, once a month or less __frequently, at least once a week
appetite loss	__rarely __occasionally, once a month or less __frequently, at least once a week
eating disorder	__rarely __occasionally, once a month or less __frequently, at least once a week
tired and sleepy after eating	__rarely __occasionally, once a month or less __frequently, at least once a week
wake up between 1 A.M. and 3 A.M.	__rarely __occasionally, once a month or less __frequently, at least once a week
	Score: ____

	Type 2: Summer
appearance:	*pale skin with frequently flushed cheeks, nose is bulbous and red, forehead is lined*
emotional hallmarks:	*excessive giddiness and/or inappropriate laughter*
flat or ridged fingernails	__rarely __occasionally, once a month or less __frequently, at least once a week
fingernails that chip or crack easily	__rarely __occasionally, once a month or less __frequently, at least once a week
skin beneath fingernails is blue or white, not pink	__rarely __occasionally, once a month or less __frequently, at least once a week
dry, itchy rashes or eczema	__rarely __occasionally, once a month or less __frequently, at least once a week
tongue is pale, crated, or red tipped	__rarely __occasionally, once a month or less __frequently, at least once a week
swelling around the ankles or shinbone	__rarely __occasionally, once a month or less __frequently, at least once a week
circulatory problems, like cold hands and feet	__rarely __occasionally, once a month or less __frequently, at least once a week
canker sores	__rarely __occasionally, once a month or less __frequently, at least once a week
angina, shortness of breath, or chest pains after doing minimal physical exertion	__rarely __occasionally, once a month or less __frequently, at least once a week
slow, irregular pulse	__rarely __occasionally, once a month or less __frequently, at least once a week
irregular or rapid heartbeat	__rarely __occasionally, once a month or less __frequently, at least once a week
problems with lymphatic circulation	__rarely __occasionally, once a month or less __frequently, at least once a week
numbness or tingling, generally in left arm or hand	__rarely __occasionally, once a month or less __frequently, at least once a week
food allergies	__rarely __occasionally, once a month or less __frequently, at least once a week

Continued

	Type 2: Summer, continued
constipation or diarrhea	__rarely __occasionally, once a month or less __frequently, at least once a week
bloating, belching, embarrassing flatulence after eating	__rarely __occasionally, once a month or less __frequently, at least once a week
severe heartburn	__rarely __occasionally, once a month or less __frequently, at least once a week
halitosis	__rarely __occasionally, once a month or less __frequently, at least once a week
chronic headaches, colds, and flus	__rarely __occasionally, once a month or less __frequently, at least once a week
not much appetite for meat or other protein	__rarely __occasionally, once a month or less __frequently, at least once a week
tired after eating	__rarely __occasionally, once a month or less __frequently, at least once a week
anemia	__rarely __occasionally, once a month or less __frequently, at least once a week
nausea	__rarely __occasionally, once a month or less __frequently, at least once a week
	Score: ____

	Type 3: Autumn
appearance:	*dry, dehydrated, blotchy skin with either a sunken chest or inflated chest, out of proportion for size; breakouts or broken vessels on cheeks and upper forehead*
emotional hallmarks:	*prolonged or unresolved grief leading to introspection and pensiveness*
dryness of skin, hair, scalp, throat, and nose	__rarely __occasionally, once a month or less __frequently, at least once a week
dry, cracked nails and lips	__rarely __occasionally, once a month or less __frequently, at least once a week
delicate, thin skin	__rarely __occasionally, once a month or less __frequently, at least once a week

	Type 3: Autumn, continued
wrinkling or shriveling of skin	__rarely __occasionally, once a month or less __frequently, at least once a week
bruises that don't heal	__rarely __occasionally, once a month or less __frequently, at least once a week
skin problems such as rashes, acne, eczema, or psoriasis	__rarely __occasionally, once a month or less __frequently, at least once a week
sinus headaches, rhinitis, or dry mucus membranes	__rarely __occasionally, once a month or less __frequently, at least once a week
problems with elimination	__rarely __occasionally, once a month or less __frequently, at least once a week
colitis or diverticulitis	__rarely __occasionally, once a month or less __frequently, at least once a week
constipation	__rarely __occasionally, once a month or less __frequently, at least once a week
diarrhea	__rarely __occasionally, once a month or less __frequently, at least once a week
more than 3 bowel movements per day	__rarely __occasionally, once a month or less __frequently, at least once a week
long, thin stools	__rarely __occasionally, once a month or less __frequently, at least once a week
foul-smelling stools	__rarely __occasionally, once a month or less __frequently, at least once a week
stools with undigested food particles	__rarely __occasionally, once a month or less __frequently, at least once a week
dry cough	__rarely __occasionally, once a month or less __frequently, at least once a week
shortness of breath	__rarely __occasionally, once a month or less __frequently, at least once a week
respiratory disorders such as asthma or bronchitis	__rarely __occasionally, once a month or less __frequently, at least once a week
wheezing	__rarely __occasionally, once a month or less __frequently, at least once a week
lack of perspiration	__rarely __occasionally, once a month or less __frequently, at least once a week

Continued

	Type 3: Autumn, continued
problems with lubrication and hydration	__rarely __occasionally, once a month or less __frequently, at least once a week
arthritis-like symptoms	__rarely __occasionally, once a month or less __frequently, at least once a week
aches and pains in joints	__rarely __occasionally, once a month or less __frequently, at least once a week
systematic yeast infections	__rarely __occasionally, once a month or less __frequently, at least once a week
	Score: ____

	Type 4: Winter
appearance:	*bluish discoloration or dark circles around the eyes, puffiness under eyes is prominent with large or misshapen ears*
emotional hallmarks:	*unresolved or ongoing fear*
dark pigmentation, freckles, or spots on face or back of hands	__rarely __occasionally, once a month or less __frequently, at least once a week
thinning or too-thick hair	__rarely __occasionally, once a month or less __frequently, at least once a week
loss of pubic or scalp hair	__rarely __occasionally, once a month or less __frequently, at least once a week
loss of hearing	__rarely __occasionally, once a month or less __frequently, at least once a week
prematurely gray, thin hair and wrinkled skin	__rarely __occasionally, once a month or less __frequently, at least once a week
weak bones, teeth, or joints, especially the knees and lower back	__rarely __occasionally, once a month or less __frequently, at least once a week
infertility or lack of sex drive; frigidity or impotence	__rarely __occasionally, once a month or less __frequently, at least once a week
weight gain	__rarely __occasionally, once a month or less __frequently, at least once a week

	Type 4: Winter, continued
extremely sensitive to light, wearing sunglasses much of the time	__rarely __occasionally, once a month or less __frequently, at least once a week
craving salt or addicted to sweets	__rarely __occasionally, once a month or less __frequently, at least once a week
light-headed feeling when you stand up too quickly	__rarely __occasionally, once a month or less __frequently, at least once a week
frequent pain or weakness in the knees or lower back	__rarely __occasionally, once a month or less __frequently, at least once a week
low blood pressure	__rarely __occasionally, once a month or less __frequently, at least once a week
low stamina	__rarely __occasionally, once a month or less __frequently, at least once a week
chronic fatigue	__rarely __occasionally, once a month or less __frequently, at least once a week
allergies, asthma, or hay fever	__rarely __occasionally, once a month or less __frequently, at least once a week
inability to deal with stress	__rarely __occasionally, once a month or less __frequently, at least once a week
difficulty in waking up and getting going in morning	__rarely __occasionally, once a month or less __frequently, at least once a week
	Score: ____

Type 1. If your highest score shows that you are a type 1, then spring (when the liver and gallbladder are the special cleansing organs) is the season when the majority of your symptoms will manifest. Although many of your beauty and health symptoms may also occur in other seasons of the year to a lesser degree, they will be magnified in the springtime.

Type 2. If you highest score shows that you are a type 2 , then summer (when the heart and small intestine are the special cleansing organs) is the season when the majority of your symptoms will manifest.

Type 3. If your highest score shows that you are a type 3, then autumn (when the lungs and large intestine are your special cleansing organs) is the season when the majority of your symptoms will manifest.

Type 4. If your highest score shows that you are a type 4, then winter (when the kidneys and adrenal glands are your special cleansing organs and glands) is the season when the majority of your symptoms will manifest.

Overall Score Results. Now add together the score from each of the four types for an overall score. If your grand total is:

- 30–58, then your symptoms reflect mild toxicity, and you should do each seasonal detox for the minimum of three days.

- 59–109 and above, then your symptoms reflect high toxicity, and you should do each seasonal detox for up to two weeks. I highly suggest that you also follow the exercises of the season and the supportive detox treatments.

You're probably beginning to see how your beauty problems aren't a curse but are the result of inner imbalances. Your body does not lie. Beauty is sabotaged by toxic overload and is further compromised by hormonal shifts as we get older. But now you have the answer at your fingertips.

With these fundamentals in hand, you're all set to embark on the Living Beauty Detox Diet program outlined in the next chapter for a more energetic, beautiful you. Remember that you can start the plan at any point. So turn to the time of year you're in now, and begin the program specifically designed for that season.

4

Spring Seasonal Detox Diet

To every thing there is a season,
and a time to every purpose under the heaven.
ECCLESIASTES 3:1

Cleansing and creating a lifestyle in harmony with the body's natural detoxification cycles can help fortify your well-being, season in and season out. The Living Beauty Detox Diet taps into nature's wondrous system of balance by using foods, healing teas, herbs, and spices to balance your body's energy, cooling it down in spring and summer and firing it up in autumn and winter. This unique cleansing, purifying program rests on the principles of Traditional Chinese Medicine, which links the seasons with certain organs. The seasons, which last approximately three months each, have their own rhythm and character, bringing with them temperature and weather changes as well as different lengths of daylight, all of which affect your health. After you read about each of these detoxifying organs in the next section, you'll gain a better understanding of why some of the symptoms listed in the Living Beauty Cleansing Questionnaire in chapter 3 manifest themselves at certain times of the year. You'll also start to see how you can take a proactive approach to better health and beauty at the same time.

A Symptom for All Seasons

Beth, a thirty-seven-year-old marketing executive, had been seeing me intermittently for about two years to get herself back on track for weight loss. I put her on my Two-Week Fat Flush program—which is covered in great detail in *Beyond Pritikin*—because of the overwhelming success my clients and readers have had with the plan for well over a decade. (A copy of this diet appears in the Appendix, although it is best used as part of the larger Beyond Pritikin program.) True to form, Beth lost ten pounds in two weeks and a good four to six inches around her waist and hips. Although she was ecstatic about her weight loss and loss of inches, I began noticing a pattern of symptoms unfolding as she came under more stress from her new executive position. Like clockwork, she was waking up between 1 A.M. and 3 A.M. every night. For the first time in her adult life, Beth had to deal with acne, which was even more stressful since she felt looking good was critical for her position.

Beth was coming in approximately once every three months to see me. As I started noting her symptoms in her chart, many were coinciding with the changing seasons. During the spring, her face was oilier, her perimenopausal symptoms (irritability, moodiness, and a short fuse) soared, and her eyes became itchy and red with frequent styes. Every summer, Beth was plagued with heart palpitations, chronic headaches, and a bloated feeling after meals. She also seemed to be emotionally more giddy and highly excitable during that time of year. By the time autumn arrived, she was having to contend with a persistent dry cough, cracked nails, achy joints, bouts of constipation, sinusitis, and a sudden onset of allergies never before experienced. And she would also become more withdrawn during autumn. In winter, Beth would invariably complain of lethargy and would battle depression.

The Two-Week Fat Flush had been successful for Beth's weight loss but obviously wasn't enough for combating these other, typically seasonal, symptoms. Since she did so well on the Fat Flush program and had sufficient energy to maintain her demanding work schedule while following the diet, I decided to augment the program with specific elements (seasonal foods, healing teas, specialty herbs, and powerhouse spices) that I knew were important for particular organs needing additional support at certain times of the year. I also knew this approach would enhance Beth's immunity by providing the necessary factors for thorough cleansing and rebuilding.

Based upon the changing needs of spring, summer, autumn, and winter, Beth's cleansing program would mirror those changes. Depending upon the season, she would take special therapeutic and beautifying oils (like flaxseed in spring, olive oil in summer, or sesame oil in winter) every day to rev up her metabolism and to lubricate her system, making elimination more efficient. Her meals were planned in accordance with seasonally available fresh produce that emphasized sulfur-rich cruciferous vegetables (like cabbage, broccoli, cauliflower, and brussels sprouts) especially critical to the cleansing process. She also included organic lean proteins—lighter fish and poultry in the warm weather and heavier meats in the autumn and winter—at every meal to maintain level blood sugar and to provide the detoxifying amino acid glutathione for her system.

No matter what the season of the year, each morning when she woke up and every night before going to bed, Beth began and ended the day by boosting detoxification. She took a special elixir containing unsweetened cranberry juice (for urinary tract health and pH balance) and an organic green superfood containing enzymes and antioxidant-rich grasses, algae, vegetables, and seeds that provided all the nutrients necessary for cleansing and supporting the detoxification pathways. A high-fiber supplement also was included to make sure her GI tract was continuously losing accumulated wastes and preventing the absorption of new toxins.

Twice a day Beth began to drink herbal teas known to target the organ of the season (like dandelion for liver cleansing in spring or fenugreek for respiratory health in autumn) as well as plenty of filtered water each day to ensure normal bowel and kidney function so her body could rid itself of wastes as well as stored "toxic" fat.

After each seasonal detox, Beth was back, excited about looking and feeling better than ever. No more perimenopausal irritability and anxiety. She had more energy, her skin had a radiant glow, her fingernails were strong and healthy looking, her hair had a wonderful sheen, and her health had improved dramatically.

Because of Beth's success, I decided to share the seasonal detox plans I devised for her with my other clients. These detox programs became the foundation to the Living Beauty Detox Diet outlined in this and the next three chapters. This simple but vital plan marks the cornerstone of discerning nutrition, better health, and living beauty through complete body purification.

As you begin your journey to a new you with the Living Beauty Detox Diet, keep in mind your season type indicated by the Living Beauty Cleansing Questionnaire in chapter 3. Take special care of yourself during that time of year by using the special supplemental herbs suggested for your season.

The Living Beauty Detox Diet for Spring

Spring, beginning with the spring solstice on March 20 or 21, heralds a time of beginning, planting, and watering. It's characterized by recreation, rejuvenation, and regeneration. All of nature awakens, impressing you with its spark and radiance. You feel alive, inspired. And you're ready to experience Mother Earth's renewal to its fullest, realizing that it's time to whisk away the old and usher in the new. So you turn careful attention to your liver and gallbladder.

Giving your liver special nurturing during the spring helps you attain better health and beauty. This program, specifically designed for this time of year, will help nourish your liver, regenerate cells and tissue, support the purification of the blood, and energize and soothe your nervous system.

Healing Tea, Herbs, and Spices for Spring

Dandelion root tea is the premier springtime herbal tea because it has a long history of gentle effective liver cleansing and decongesting. It's known as a primary liver tonic and offers more nutritional value than most vegetables. Dandelion root also helps alleviate liver inflammation and congestion by stimulating bile. Other liver-protecting herbs include gentian root, which stimulates the gallbladder to increase secretion and flush out bacteria; milk thistle, which protects and regenerates the liver by preventing free-radical damage through its potent antioxidant properties found in the active component known as silymarin; yellow dock, which acts as a liver purifier and toner through cleansing the bloodstream; and Oregon grape root, which is helpful in liver-connected skin conditions such as acne and psoriasis. Chlorophyll-rich spices like dill, mint, tarragon, and thyme are time-honored detoxifiers that nourish and purify the bloodstream while assisting the body in the digestive process. The juices from both fresh lemons and limes, natural diuretics, are also included in the spring detox plan because of their antiseptic, germicidal, and mucus-eliminating properties. They have been used for centuries as liver toners.

Following the Spring Detox Plan

Spring is the time to emphasize lots of fresh vegetables, especially purifying, dark green, leafy ones like kale and parsley, which are high in chlorophyll. For the spring detox plan (whether you stay on it for three days or two weeks, depending on your results from the Living Beauty Cleansing Questionnaire in chapter 3), the foods to be consumed for breakfast, lunch, and dinner should be chosen from the following food groups only. You can individualize the spring menu plans to suit your own taste preferences by substituting one food for another from the same food group categories listed below.

If you cannot locate organic produce, remember that the daily use of the Living Beauty Elixir with its green superfood key component can provide the concentrated antioxidants, vitamins, minerals, and enzymes that may be missing from the nonorganic sources. The following list is restricted to whole natural foods eaten without salt, vinegar, soy sauce, mustard, and most additional herbs and spices. The exceptions, of course, are the cleansing spring spices of dill, mint, parsley, rosemary, tarragon, and thyme, the cleansing juices of fresh lemon and lime, plus the spring tea, dandelion root. You may use natural, unsalted chicken broth and beef broth for special dishes on the menu plans if you need more liquids for basting or sautéing than the limit of 2 tablespoons of oil.

	Spring Detox Plan Protocol
Oil	1 tablespoon organic lignan-rich flaxseed oil twice daily
Lean Protein	(at least 8 ounces per day) All varieties of eggs, fish, lamb, poultry, veal, pheasant, and quail
Vegetables	Unlimited, raw or steamed, low glycemic. Choose from high-fiber selections: artichokes, asparagus, bamboo shoots, beans (green, Italian, and wax), broccoli, brussels spouts, cabbage (bok choy, Chinese, green, or red), celery, cauliflower, cucumbers, eggplant, escarole, greens (arugula, Belgian endive, butterleaf of bib, dandelion, escarole, kale, kohlrabi, mustard greens, parsley, radicchio, romaine, spinach, and watercress), horseradish, onions (Bermuda, chives, green, leeks, scallions, shallots), peppers (green, red, and yellow), sprouts (clover, mung bean, radish, and sunflower), squash (crookneck, Italian, patty pan, scallop, yellow, or zucchini), tomatoes, and water chestnuts.
Fruits	2 whole portions daily. Choose from 1 small apple (Golden Delicious, Red Delicious, Macintosh, Newton, Pippin, Rome Beauty, or Granny Smith); ½ small avocado; 2 medium apricots, ½ grapefruit; I medium nectarine; 1 orange; 2 small plums; or 1½ cups strawberries.
Filtered Water	8 glasses a day to rid the body of waste, keep tissues moist, and lubricate the system
With or Between Meals	Take 1 cup of dandelion root tea daily.
Breakfast and Dinner (optional)	Take a liver-supporting supplement containing one or more of the following herbs: gentian root, yellow dock, milk thistle, and Oregon grape root. Follow directions on the label.

Here are some sample days of the Spring Detox Plan:

	Sample Day One Spring Detox Plan
Upon Arising	Living Beauty Elixir with 2 high-fiber supplements
	2 eight-ounce glasses of water
Before Breakfast	1 cup dandelion root tea
Breakfast	½ grapefruit
	2 soft-boiled or hard-boiled eggs
	Steamed fresh kale and red bell peppers with dash of thyme
Midmorning	2 eight-ounce glasses of water
Lunch	4 ounces broiled spring lamb patty with ⅛ teaspoon rosemary
	Super Cleansing Salad (with watercress, tomatoes, radish, and mung bean sprouts)
	Dressing of 1 tablespoon flaxseed oil, fresh lemon juice, and chives
Midafternoon	2 eight-ounce glasses of water
4 P.M.	1½ cups strawberries
Dinner	4 ounces poached fresh salmon with dill
	Spring Beauty Salad Bowl (with minced parsley, chopped tomatoes, and diced scallions with 1tablespoon flaxseed oil, fresh lime juice, and ½ teaspoon mint)
	Steamed brussels sprouts
	1 cup dandelion root tea
Midevening	Living Beauty Elixir with 2 high-fiber supplements
	2 eight-ounce glasses of water

	Sample Day Two Spring Detox Plan
Upon Arising	Living Beauty Elixir with 2 high-fiber supplements
	2 eight-ounce glasses of water

Continued

	Sample Day Two Spring Detox Plan, continued
Before Breakfast	1 cup dandelion root tea
Breakfast	1 orange
	2 hard-boiled eggs with fresh parsley
	Tomato slices with tarragon
Midmorning	2 eight-ounce glasses of water
Lunch	Avocado salad with ½ small avocado, lime juice, cucumbers, spring greens, tomatoes, and shallots with 1 tablespoon flaxseed oil
Midafternoon	2 eight-ounce glasses of water
4 P.M.	1 Granny Smith apple
Dinner	4 ounces broiled lamb chop with lemon juice, parsley, rosemary, and thyme
	Mixed Green Salad
	Steamed artichoke with 1 tablespoon flaxseed oil
	1 cup dandelion root tea
Midevening	Living Beauty Elixir with 2 high-fiber supplements
	2 eight-ounce glasses of water

	Sample Day Three Spring Detox Plan
Upon Arising	Living Beauty Elixir with 2 high-fiber supplements
	2 eight-ounce glasses of water
Before Breakfast	1 cup dandelion root tea
Breakfast	½ grapefruit
	Spring Rainbow Eggs (with 2 poached eggs on zucchini, yellow squash, and red peppers)
Midmorning	2 eight-ounce glasses of water

	Sample Day Three Spring Detox Plan, continued
Lunch	4 ounces baked chicken breast with tarragon
	Spring vegetable medley
	Dressing of 1 tablespoon flaxseed oil, lemon juice, and dill
Midafternoon	2 eight-ounce glasses of water
4 P.M.	2 medium apricots
Dinner	4 ounces veal strips with lemon juice
	Mixed sprout salad with 1 tablespoon flaxseed oil and lemon juice with parsley and mint
	Steamed asparagus and string beans
	1 cup dandelion root tea
Midevening	Living Beauty Elixir with 2 high-fiber supplements
	2 eight-ounce glasses of water

Spring Maintenance Plan

If you wish to continue cleansing up to two weeks, based upon your results of the Living Beauty Cleansing Questionnaire in chapter 3, then continue to use the basic Spring Detox plan protocol.

For those of you who are ready to enjoy all of spring's fresh offerings and still maintain your cleansing results, you now may add additional high-fiber and purifying foods back into your eating plan. I do suggest, however, that at least once a day you continue with spring's dandelion root tea and the Living Beauty Elixir. You may include foods from the fiber-rich, low-glycemic or slow-acting starch family (vegetables and beans), beginning with one serving at a time in the amounts listed below. Weight permitting, you can ultimately include up to four servings a day from each of the starch selections.

In addition, you can include 1–2 servings of yogurt or cottage cheese a day, which is good for a light lunch or a snack. Do keep in mind, however, that because of dairy's possible allergic component as well as the magnesium-calcium interaction, you should limit your intake of high-calcium dairy products. I recommend no more than 2 portions a day of either yogurt or cottage cheese. These dairy products are the easiest to digest and have healing properties because they are "cultured." They provide the friendly bacteria, which helps keep the system free from pathogenic bacteria, virus, and parasites.

The Spring Starchy Vegetables Selection

One serving of starchy vegetables equals any one of the following:

Beets—1 cup

Burdock root (raw)—½ cup

Corn—½ cup

Sweet peas—½ cup

Potato—½ medium

The Spring Beans Selection

One serving of beans equals any one of the following:

Fava beans—½ cup

Green split peas—½ cup

Lentils—½ cup

The Spring Dairy Selection

One serving of dairy equals any one of the following:

Goat milk or whole milk yogurt—1 cup

Whole or 2% cottage cheese—½ cup

Spring Maintenance Menu Plan

Here is a sample day of the Spring Maintenance Menu Plan:

	Sample Day Spring Maintenance Plan
Upon Arising	Living Beauty Elixir with 2 high-fiber supplements
	2 eight-ounce glasses of water
Before Breakfast	1 cup dandelion root tea
Breakfast	2 medium apricots
	Minty Spring Cottage Cheese (with ½ cup 2% cottage cheese, ½ teaspoon mint, and 1 tablespoon flaxseed oil)
Midmorning	2 eight-ounce glasses of water
Lunch	2 hard-boiled eggs
	Mixed spring greens with lemon juice and tarragon
	½ cup new baby potatoes with minced parsley and onions, drizzled with ½ tablespoon flaxseed oil
Midafternoon	2 eight-ounce glasses of water
4 P.M.	½ small avocado with lime juice
Dinner	4 ounces grilled spring lamb
	Baby vegetable mélange of asparagus tips, mung bean, radish, and sunflower sprouts
	½ cup sweet peas, ½ tablespoon flaxseed oil, dash of thyme
Midevening	2 eight-ounce glasses of water

Spring into Health—Get Going with Exercise!

After a sedentary winter, many people can be carrying around as much as ten pounds of toxic wastes. Some combination of cardiovascular, strength-building, and flexibility exercises can be enjoyed during your seasonal detox program and thereafter during the entire season. Now that the weather is changing, be sure to balance your exercise between indoor and outdoor activity. However, it is distinctly more beneficial to exercise outside for the invigorating fresh air. Remember also that sunlight provides bone-building Vitamin D and also provides stimulation to the optic nerve, which tones every gland in the body.

The best cardiovascular exercises for those of you in your teens, twenties, thirties, forties, fifties, and above during the spring detox period and beyond include brisk walking, treadmills, jogging, tennis, volleyball, badminton, and low-impact aerobic dancing for three to four days a week for at least thirty minutes each day. Being outside in the fresh air will oxygenate your system and help the cleansing process. For women in their thirties, forties, fifties, and above, do include some strength training at least twice a week for about forty-five minutes. Women with very low bone density should concentrate on swimming, walking in water, water aerobics, or cycling rather than impact activities, which can increase fracture risk. Each age group can benefit from daily stretching exercises for enhanced flexibility. Build up gradually.

Springtime Liver/Gallbladder–Supporting Treatments During Detox and Beyond

Castor Oil Pack

Since ancient times, castor oil has been used as healing oil for a variety of maladies but particularly for those related to the liver and gallbladder. Castor oil is believed to be able to penetrate deeply—as much as four inches—into the body. At a 1992 Conference of the American Association of Naturopathic Physicians in Tempe, Arizona, it was reported that daily use of castor oil packs resulted in a normalizing effect of liver enzymes and greater well-being and energy among the research participants.

I frequently use castor oil packs as a detox therapy to stimulate the liver and gallbladder and to draw out toxins from the body. My clients report a remarkable sense of well-being and tranquillity while applying the castor oil pack. Since the emotion of anger is so closely tied to the liver, you may find that angry feeling you have buried start to resurface. Stay with your feelings, and try to channel them constructively. When I start to experience such feelings, I try to transform them into forgiveness, first to myself and then to others.

You will need three things: 100 percent pure, cold-pressed castor oil; wool (not cotton) flannel; and a heating pad.

1. Fold the wool flannel into three or four layers, and soak it with castor oil.

2. Put the flannel in a baking dish and heat it slowly in the oven until it becomes hot, but not hot enough to scald or injure your skin.

3. Rub castor oil on your stomach, lie down, and place the hot flannel on top of your stomach.

4. Seal off the flannel with plastic wrap.

5. Cover with a heating pad for one hour, keeping the flannel as hot as safely and comfortably possible.

When you finish, wash the oil from your stomach. You can keep the oil-soaked flannel sealed in a glass container until further use, since castor oil does not become rancid as quickly as many other oils. During the initial detox period, I recommend that you use the castor oil pack once a day for three successive days, take three days off, and then use it for another three successive days. You can safely continue this regimen throughout the spring season, especially if you suffer from liver-based symptoms like eye problems; tension between your shoulders; PMS, peri-menopausal, and menopausal irritability, mood swings, bloating, tender breasts, hot flashes, and anxiety.

5

Summer Seasonal Detox Diet

Summertime . . . and the livin' is easy.
PORGY AND BESS

The summer solstice kicks off the beginning of the season on the longest day of the year, which falls on June 21. This is the season where the sun reaches its highest point in the sky and provides more daylight hours than any other time of year. Summer, powered by its fiery element, sets the stage for energy, vitality, growth, and maturing. Flowers bloom, fruits and vegetables become plentiful, vegetation flourishes. Your body's innate wisdom is somehow preparing you for a season packed with activities. You may even find yourself staying outdoors more, playing sports, and enjoying picnics, walks, and campouts with family and friends. This natural cycle of motion creates the perfect season to focus on your heart and small intestine.

With every pulse, your heart helps pump vital nutrients to every sector of the body, working in tandem with the liver, the regulator of circulation. The steady beat of your heart helps control circulation so the detoxification process receives its proper nourishment. Highly active in summer, this four-chambered muscle—the strongest muscle in your body—provides the energy and messages needed to stimulate organs so they work in harmony. The heart pumps approximately 3,000 gallons of blood daily to the lungs, where it absorbs oxygen. Then the blood returns to the heart, where it is pumped out to the body, carrying oxygen and vital nutrients. Like a long-lasting battery, your heart can keep going and going as long as it has enough oxygen. But when your lungs are impaired or your liver is overly stressed, problems arise. In fact, if your liver isn't functioning normally, the blood supply—up to 70 percent of it—can become blocked and thwart the circulation and oxygen-fueling process.

You already know that smoking and high cholesterol can endanger your heart's functions. However, a number of other factors can negatively affect the heart, such as your emotions. Every time you become tense, the rate and rhythm of your heart are affected, which disturbs the blood and oxygen flow. And that causes the blood vessels in your wrists and ankles to become constricted; consequently, your hands and feet feel cold. In time, a lowered supply of oxygen to your heart can produce secondary symptoms such as angina; heart palpitations, irregular beats, and possibly a heart attack can manifest.

Escalated levels of a potentially toxic amino acid called homocysteine can also make you a likely candidate for cardiovascular disease by damaging blood vessels and contributing to plaque buildup. As a matter of fact, having a higher-than-normal amount of homocysteine in your body can become so dangerous that it actually equals the dangers that smoking and high cholesterol levels have on your heart, according to a *New England Journal of Medicine* study done in 1997. Homocysteine is the metabolic byproduct of a methionine breakdown, an amino acid found in animal protein. In ideal functions, homocysteine passes through a detoxification process known as methylation, where it is converted to the nontoxic amino acid cysteine. But this process can operate properly only if vitamins B_{12}, B_6, and folic acid are readily available. Having low amounts of these critical B vitamins (particularly B_{12}, which is mandatory for the conversion process and the production of folic acid), consuming an overabundance of animal protein (meat, eggs, dairy), and drinking a lot of coffee all can aggravate normal functions and cause homocysteine levels to climb. The result may be the all-too-familiar forgetfulness, cloudy thinking, or other Alzheimer's-like symptoms frequently associated with growing old. A 1996 Physician's Health Study conducted at Harvard reported that among the 271 men in the group, 95 percent of those who suffered heart attacks also had elevated homocysteine levels.

According to Traditional Chinese Medicine, when the "fire" of your heart becomes out of balance because impaired kidneys (the "water" element) are not keeping it cooled, your heart produces hot flashes, night sweats, and palpitations. You also become uneasy, feeling irritable and restlessness and experiencing insomnia and nightmares. Your skin may appear reddish, your cheeks are often flushed, and you may have a bulbous or red nose.

How's your heart? You might want to check out the color and texture of your tongue in a mirror. According to Traditional Chinese Medicine, the color of the tongue reflects the health of the heart. What you want to see is a moist, pink-colored tongue. Paleness could indicate anemia, and a coated tongue could suggest digestive problems. (Smokers typically will have a yellowish tongue.) You might also want to take a look at your body color, especially your fingertips and beneath your fingernails. Is the color red, pink, blue, or perhaps white? And take note if you have any swelling around the ankles or shinbone, which could suggest poor circulation, too much salt, or fluid retention.

Summer is also the time to focus on your small intestine, another important component of the detox process. The vital nutrients upon which detoxification depends are made available to your body through your small intestine. Linking the stomach to the large intestine, your twenty-three-foot-long small intestine changes the food you eat into useful elements such as glucose, fatty acids, and the much-needed amino acids, with help from enzymes in the pancreas and bile from the liver and gallbladder. The small intestine digests and absorbs nutrients, then ships them off to the bloodstream, where they are carried to the liver. There they are either used or stored in the form of glycogen, which reverts to the original substances (glucose, fatty acids, or amino acids) when needed to nourish the whole system. Keeping the small intestine clear is vital for the overall health of the body. If your intestinal lining becomes coated with mucus, nutrient absorption is greatly diminished, which zaps your immune system functions and opens the door to food allergies and a number of illnesses as well as fatigue from a rise in white blood cell production. Having an impaired digestive tract causes the loss of essential building blocks, resulting in poor-quality skin, hair, and nails, and indigestion with its accompanying bloating, excess gas, stomach pain, and constipation. In fact, your small intestines are the critical stop for digestion and good health. But to function normally, your digestive system (which stretches from your lips to your anus) needs the enzyme ptyalin (which is in saliva); hydrochloric acid (HCL), which is produced in the stomach; and pancreatic enzymes.

Here's how the digestive process works to keep your system in balance. In the first stage of the digestive process, your food enters the upper part of the stomach. It may stay there for approximately one hour while your body manufactures the acid needed to stimulate enzymes so it can digest protein. Then the second stage begins as the food causes the walls of your stomach to swell. Your stomach's parietal cells obtain sufficient amounts of HCL from the blood so the stomach has a pH that is highly acidic. The partially digested food moves down into the lower part of your stomach, where pepsin (an enzyme) is secreted to help with the metabolic breakdown of dietary protein. Meanwhile, HCL stimulates the pepsin and continues to do its job maintaining the acidity, which in turn helps the pepsin complete its duties of breaking down the protein. HCL also helps in the third stage by stimulating the pancreas so it manufactures the enzymes needed for this phase of digestion. At this point in the process, the partially digested food slips through the pyloric valve, the opening to your intestines, and enters the alkaline pH of your small intestine. Bicarbonate, pancreatic enzymes (protease, amylase, and lipase), and bile also move into the intestine to help digest the food more completely.

As you may have noticed, HCL plays a critical role in the entire process. This digestive acid might be considered one of the most important chemicals in your body, since it helps to metabolize protein, minerals, calcium, and iron. When HCL is missing, protein can't be broken down properly into amino acids, hindering the maintenance and building of muscles. These nonmetabolized proteins begin to decay and enter the bloodstream. Now a toxic waste, the putrefied proteins make their way throughout your system, placing more stress on your lungs, kidneys, skin, and bowels. Putrefaction can be a major underlying cause of body odors, gas, halitosis, and malodorous urine and stools.

Since two of the minerals most vital to females, iron and calcium, require an acid medium, low HCL production reduces your body's digestion and therefore use and absorption of these minerals. Consequently, iron doesn't get into your blood cells, making your skin look devitalized, pale and pasty. You feel tired, run-down, or anemic. Calcium can no longer be absorbed into your system to create lovely teeth and beautiful, strong bones; instead, it builds up in the soft tissues, where it can result in arthritis and atherosclerosis. Lacking calcium may also mean having high sodium levels and low potassium levels, which throws off the rhythm of your systems since potassium is needed for your heartbeat.

But what exactly causes HCL levels to plummet? Well, forget the old notion that it only happens to elderly people whose stomachs no longer produce sufficient levels of HCL. Today, having an HCL deficiency can happen to anyone regardless of age, including babies. Topping the list of causes are emotional tension and diet. Which means if you're upset, highly stressed, continually on the go, or quarreling during meals, you could be setting yourself up for HCL trouble. The absence of vital nutrients, such as vitamins B_1 (thiamin), B_2 (riboflavin), or B_6 (pyridoxine), niacin, choline, folic acid, or protein, could also instigate an HCL deficiency. And if you tend to drink liquids with your meals, consume lots of carbonated beverages, even carbonated mineral waters, or eat your meals hurriedly or forget to chew your food sufficiently, you could have reduced HCL levels.

When your HCL production is low, the opening to your small intestine (called the pylorus) doesn't function normally, causing lowered levels of bile and a slow-moving bowel. And that results in constipation, which clearly begins in the intestine. The bile that was supposed to be in the small intestine ends up in the liver. Your pancreas becomes taxed, and soon pancreatitis occurs. Like a set of well-stacked dominoes, a low HCL production affects the liver, gallbladder, and pancreas, which all lead to indigestion, gas, belching, bloating, constipation, diarrhea, and vomiting. When you're HCL deficient, you may look pale or drawn, and you even age more quickly.

People often mistakenly label their indigestion as having too much acid in their stomachs, and they try to correct the problem with antacids. However, they may actually have too little acid, in other words, an HCL deficiency. You may also want to purchase an HCL-with-pepsin tablet or capsule (10 grains HCL to 2 grains pepsin), available in most health food stores. Since the symptoms for an excess HCL production can mirror those of having too little, you need to be cautious. If that gaseous or lumpy feeling disappears after taking an HCL tablet during a protein meal, then you know it was HCL related.

The Living Beauty Detox Diet for Summer

Enjoying the energy of the season will be easier as you follow the Living Beauty Detox Diet program for summer. You'll not only provide your heart and small intestines the care they need, but you will also be mapping out a foundation for well-being and enhanced beauty.

Healing Tea, Herbs, and Spices for Summer

Rose hips tea is the summertime herbal tea of choice because it is an exceptionally high source of vitamin C and bioflavonoids, which are important for a healthy heart, blood vessels, circulation, immunity, and the integrity of the GI tract's mucosal lining. Other heart-protecting herbs include hawthorn berries, which lower high blood pressure, normalize low blood pressure, and can treat angina, irregular heartbeat, and arterial spasm; cayenne pepper, which is a heart stimulant and blood cleanser known for its ability to regulate circulation; fennel seed, which relieves gas and GI tract spasms and is good for overacidity; and licorice root, which helps to cleanse the GI tract, normalize inflammatory intestinal disorders, and promote intestinal health by stimulating protective mucus secretion for the irritated and porous mucosal lining of the digestive tract.

Garlic, summer's stinking rose, improves circulation, normalizes high and low blood pressure, and lowers blood lipid levels while helping to treat arteriosclerosis. Use cayenne, fennel seed, coriander, oregano, and garlic in your summertime cooking to further support your heart and small intestines. As in the spring plan, both cleansing and refreshing lemon and lime juices can be used as seasonings.

Because good digestion is so closely linked to allergy and autoimmune diseases, additional digestive support may be in order for those suffering from allergy or autoimmune disorders. These supplements include hydrochloric acid and pepsin; pancreatic enzymes or plant-based enzymes to prevent the toxic byproducts of impaired digestion from further damaging the intestinal lining. Follow instructions on the label. The addition of L-glutamine (500–1,000 mgs. a day between meals) is an effective amino acid to stimulate and repair the cellular lining of the small intestine.

Following the Summer Detox Plan

Summer is the time for cooling foods, especially more raw fresh fruits and fiber-rich vegetables, which not only are deliciously purifying but also are vital to eliminating the summer heat from the system. The summer sun, which induces perspiration, also helps to release toxins during this time of the year. As in spring, for the summer detox plan (whether you cleanse for the minimum three days or two weeks), pick foods for breakfast, lunch, and dinner from the food groups listed below. Remember, of course, that you can individualize the summer menu plans to suit your own taste preferences by substituting one food for another from the same food group categories.

This list is restricted to whole natural foods eaten without salt, vinegar, soy sauce, mustard, and most other herbs and spices. The exceptions are the detoxifying summer spices, cayenne, fennel seed, coriander, oregano, and garlic, and the summer tea, rose hips. You may use unsalted chicken broth and beef broth for special dishes on the menu plans if you need more liquids for basting or sautéing than the limit of 2 tablespoons of oil. You will also note that for summer I have included sauerkraut. Sauerkraut is one of the best ways I know to increase the beneficial *L. plantarum* bacteria, a powerful probiotic that destroys many toxic strains of bacteria and parasites in the gastrointestinal tract.

	Summer Detox Plan Protocol
Oils	1 tablespoon lignan-rich flaxseed oil and 1 tablespoon heart-smart virgin olive oil. Olive oil is beneficial because it has been shown to reduce LDL ("bad cholesterol") levels while keeping HDL ("good cholesterol") levels high. It is monounsaturated oil, which stands up well to the summertime heat.
Lean Protein	(at least 8 ounces per day) As in spring, all varieties of fish, water-packed tuna, water-packed sardines, water-packed salmon, eggs, lean beef, and poultry. For the light breakfasts of fruit smoothies in the summer detox plan, choose high-protein powders such as those made of lactose-free whey. The powder should yield at least 12 to 14 grams of protein per tablespoon, which approximates one ounce of animal protein. Most of these protein powders can be found in health food stores.
Vegetables	Unlimited, raw or steamed, low glycemic. Choose from high-fiber selections: broccoli, brussels sprouts, bamboo shoots, cabbage (bok choy, Chinese, green, or red), raw carrots,* cauliflower, cilantro, cucumbers, garlic, greens (arugula, Belgian endive, butterleaf of bib, dandelion, escarole, kale, kohlrabi, mustard greens, parsley, radicchio, Romaine, spinach, and watercress), hearts of palm, horseradish, jicama,† onions (Bermuda, chives, green, leeks, scallions, shallots), peppers (green, red, and yellow), salsify, squash (crookneck, Italian, patty pan, scallop, yellow, or zucchini), tomatoes. * Eat carrots raw; when cooked or juiced, the loss of the fiber makes them a starchy vegetable. † Jicama is a good source of inulin, a prebiotic or friendly undigested carbohydrate that feeds the intestinal bacteria; delicious as a crunchy, sweet snack. 3 tablespoons sauerkraut (choose health food store brands)

Continued

	Summer Detox Plan Protocol, continued
Fruits	3 whole portions daily: Choose from ½ medium banana; 1 cup berries (blackberries, blueberries, and raspberries); 1 small kiwi; 1 cup melon (cantaloupe, casaba, honeydew); ½ cup papaya; ½ medium mango; 1 medium nectarine; 1 medium peach; ¾ cup pineapple; 2 plums; 1¼ cup watermelon.
Filtered Water	8 glasses a day to rid the body of waste, keep tissues moist, and lubricate the system
With or Between Meals	Take 2 cups of rose hips tea daily.
Breakfast and Dinner (optional)	Take a heart-supporting supplement containing hawthorn berries, garlic, or cayenne.

Here are some sample days of the Summer Detox Plan:

	Sample Day One Summer Detox Plan
Upon Arising	Living Beauty Elixir with 2 high-fiber supplements 2 eight-ounce glasses of water
Before Breakfast	1 cup rose hips tea
Breakfast	Enzyme-rich Papaya-Banana Smoothie (blending ½ papaya with ½ banana with eight ounces of filtered water and 1 scoop of unflavored protein powder and 1 tablespoon flaxseed oil)
Midmorning	2 eight-ounce glasses of water
Lunch	Summer Beauty Salad Niçoise (made with 3 ounces water-packed tuna, olives, green beans, and tomatoes on Romaine lettuce with 1 tablespoon olive oil and lemon juice) 3 tablespoons sauerkraut with ¼ teaspoon fennel seeds
Midafternoon	2 eight-ounce glasses of water
4 P.M.	1 small kiwi

	Sample Day One Summer Detox Plan, continued
Dinner	3 ounces charcoal-broiled Cornish game hen with garlic cloves and pureed summer squash
	Cooling gazpacho (made with 2 tomatoes, peeled and seeded; ½ cucumber, peeled and seeded; ¼ chopped onion, ½ cup ice water blended until smooth with a dash of cayenne pepper)
	Sliced jicama with lime
	1 cup rose hips tea
Midevening	Living Beauty Elixir with 2 high-fiber supplements
	2 eight-ounce glasses of water

	Sample Day Two Summer Detox Plan
Upon Arising	Living Beauty Elixir with 2 high-fiber supplements
	2 eight-ounce glasses of water
Before Breakfast	1 cup rose hips tea
Breakfast	1 cup berries
	2 eggs scrambled with 1 tablespoon olive oil, mustard greens, onions, and dash of oregano
Midmorning	2 eight-ounce glasses of water
Lunch	Tuna-Pineapple Salad (with 4 ounces canned, flaked tuna, minced green onions, celery, and ¾ cup fresh pineapple mixed with 1 tablespoon flaxseed oil, dash of cayenne, served on summer greens)
	3 tablespoons sauerkraut with ½ teaspoon fennel seeds
Midafternoon	2 eight-ounce glasses of water
4 P.M.	2 plums

Continued

	Sample Day Two Summer Detox Plan, continued
Dinner	4 ounces lean broiled turkey burger with ⅛ teaspoon fennel
	Yellow squash, bamboo shoots, broccoli, and cauliflower
	1 cup rose hips tea
Midevening	Living Beauty Elixir with 2 high-fiber supplements
	2 eight-ounce glasses of water

	Sample Day Three Summer Detox Plan
Upon Arising	Living Beauty Elixir with 2 high-fiber supplements
	2 eight-ounce glasses of water
Before Breakfast	1 cup rose hips tea
Breakfast	Watermelon-Mango Smoothie (blending ¾ cup watermelon and ½ medium mango in 8 ounces of filtered water, 1 scoop unflavored protein powder, and 1 tablespoon flaxseed oil)
Midmorning	2 eight-ounce glasses of water
Lunch	Salmon-Cilantro Summer Salad (with 4 ounces canned flaked salmon, minced scallions, celery, cilantro, and oregano with a dash of cayenne, served on summer greens)
	Grated jicama, carrots, and cucumber salad
Midafternoon	2 eight-ounce glasses of water
4 P.M.	1 medium nectarine
Dinner	4 ounces broiled halibut brushed with 1 tablespoon olive oil, lemon juice, and garlic
	Watercress salad with lime
	Steamed chard, zucchini, and brussels sprouts
	1 cup rose hips tea

	Sample Day Three Summer Detox Plan, continued
Midevening	Living Beauty Elixir with 2 high-fiber supplements
	2 eight-ounce glasses of water

Summer Maintenance Plan

If you need to continue cleansing for up to two weeks, as indicated by your results from the Living Beauty Cleansing Questionnaire in chapter 3, then simply continue following the basic summer detox plan protocol. I do suggest, however, that at least once a day you continue with summer's rose hips tea and the Living Beauty Elixir to maintain a toxic-free system. For those of you who are ready for maintenance yet want to sustain your cleansing momentum, now you may add back certain high-fiber foods from the summer starch family (vegetables and beans), beginning with one serving at a time. Weight permitting, you can ultimately include up to four servings a day from each of the summer starch selections. In addition, you can include 1–2 servings of cooling yogurt or cottage cheese per day.

The Summer Starchy Vegetables Selection

One serving of starchy vegetables equals any one of the following:

Carrots (cooked)—1 cup

Corn—½ cup or 1 small corn-on-the-cob

Green peas—½ cup

Lima beans—½ cup

Rutabaga (raw)—¼ large

The Summer Beans Selection

One serving of beans equals any one of the following:

Garbanzos—⅓ cup

Fava beans—½ cup

Green split peas—½ cup

Lentils—⅓ cup

The Summer Dairy Selection

One serving of dairy equals any one of the following:

Plain goat-milk or cow's-milk yogurt—1 cup

Cottage cheese—½ cup

Summer Maintenance Menu Plan

Here is a sample day of the Summer Maintenance Menu Plan:

	Sample Day Summer Maintenance Plan
Upon Arising	Living Beauty Elixir with 2 high-fiber supplements
	2 eight-ounce glasses of water
Before Breakfast	1 cup rose hips tea
Breakfast	Summer Confetti Fruit Salad (with 1 cup low-fat yogurt, 2 cups mixed cantaloupe and honeydew melons, and ½ tablespoon flaxseed oil)
Midmorning	2 eight-ounce glasses of water
Lunch	4 ounces broiled red snapper with 1 tablespoon olive oil and dash of oregano
	Tomato and watercress salad
	Blanched collard and mustard greens with lemon juice
	½ cup lima beans

	Sample Day Summer Maintenance Plan, continued
Midafternoon	2 eight-ounce glasses of water
4 P.M.	1 medium peach
Dinner	4 ounces poached salmon
	Steamed Summer Vegetable Potpourri
	1 small corn-on-the-cob with ½ tablespoon flaxseed oil
	3 tablespoons sauerkraut with ½ teaspoon fennel seed
Midevening	2 eight-ounce glasses of water

Summer Exercise

In the warm weather of summer, make sure to drink even more water before exercising to replace fluids that will be lost in perspiration. The rule of thumb for total daily water consumption is a quart of water per 100 pounds of body weight. Some fitness buffs feel best when they drink a glass of water on the hour to ensure sufficient hydration of body tissue. Water is a marvelous body hydrator and will assist in keeping a steady body temperature.

If you are exercising indoors under air conditioning, try to match the air conditioning temperature as much as possible with that of the out-side so your system will not be stressed and subject to summer colds by the extreme variation in temperature.

For summer fitness and health, cotton clothing is your best bet; light-weight materials that can easily absorb perspiration and then dry quickly are advisable. Try to avoid antiperspirants, which block sweating, the body's natural cooling mechanism. This is particularly important for those women in their forties and fifties who may be experiencing hot flashes or night sweats.

For those in your teens and twenties, consider a program that in-cludes cardiovascular exercise at least three days a week for at least thirty minutes each day. Summer hiking, brisk walking, water-skiing, and rowing are great for cardiovascular health. For women in their thirties, forties, fifties, and beyond, in addition to the summer cardiovascular activities at least three to four days a week for thirty minutes each day, include strength training at least twice a week for about forty-five minutes each time. Flexibility exercises like stretching can be enjoyed on a daily basis. Remember that swimming and water aerobics are great for those of you who have some degree of osteoporosis, when extensive walking and hiking are not appropriate because of fracture risk.

Summertime Circulatory Supporting Treatments During Detox and Beyond

Rebounding and Skin Brushing

Both rebounding (bouncing on a minitrampoline) and skin brushing target the lymphatic system, a kind of secondary circulatory system, which transports all kinds of waste products from the blood to the cells. Although the lymphatic system is anatomically separate from our arteries and veins, it is nevertheless closely related. And while blood circulation has a rhythmic flow dictated by the pumping of the heart, the lymphatics are dependent upon muscle contraction to provide their flow. The lymphatic system is the garbage collection system of the body. It picks up foreign organisms and all the metabolic wastes from fats and proteins and brings them to the lymph nodes for more extensive processing. When they get overwhelmed, the nodes get inflamed, becoming swollen and painful.

When doing your summer detox program, it is a good idea to address specific lymphatic cleansing. One of the most effective ways to cleanse the lymph system is with the use of a minitrampoline, or rebounder. Simply use the minitrampoline for at least five minutes a day. Lean onto the balls of your feet, and walk in place. Since the lymph system has no pump, this exercise stimulates circulation in the lymph, which can rid the body of toxins and waste products. Stretching exercises are also effective for stimulating the lymph flow.

Skin brushing can also help stimulate the lymph. All you will need is a natural bristle brush that can be purchased from a health food store or bathhouse. Cheryl Townsley, a noted author and lifestyle counselor from Littleton, Colorado, suggests that before you start to dry-brush the skin, you should stimulate the two primary lymph ducts. These ducts can be found at the base of the collarbone (one on each side) and also in the groin area. Rub these areas for a few seconds to get the ducts opened. To skin-brush effectively, Townsley has her clients follow this procedure and brush three to six times a week. I suggest that you follow this procedure up to six times a week throughout the summer season:

1. Open ducts [to do this gently massage just below the collarbone (1st set of ducts) and in the groin area (2d set of ducts)].

2. Brush dry skin with clean, frequently washed natural bristle brush.

3. Use small, light circular motions.

4. Start close to the ducts and work outward.

5. From the waist up, brush toward the upper pair of ducts (under collarbone).

6. From the waist down, brush toward the lower pair of ducts (in groin area).

6

Autumn Seasonal Detox Diet

How sweet on this autumnal day the wild-wood fruits to gather.
WILLIAM WORDSWORTH

Beginning on September 22, the autumnal equinox signals a time of change—in weather, daylight, and temperatures. Days are shorter, the nights are cooler. As the colors of summer are stripped from the trees and quietly transformed to deep, rich hues, you're reminded that winter is nearing and you need to prepare. It's the ideal time to finish projects begun in these last two seasons, to concentrate on home and families, and to begin to slow down, storing your energy for the upcoming cold months. But you also want to head off the possible depression stemming from Seasonal Affective Disorder (SAD), so you take the time to enjoy as much natural sunlight as you safely can before the darker days of winter arrive. Emotionally, you learn to let go and open yourself up to change as you pause to reflect inward. Physically, you need to take special care of the two vital organs of this season, the lungs and large intestines.

Your lungs—along with the bronchial tubes, throat, sinuses, and nose—are equally important as another major detox pathway. They are your first line of defense against unhealthy air; they hold the key to respiration. Your lungs act as the go-between for the internal and outer environment, inhaling oxygen and exhaling carbon dioxide through their pulmonary capillaries. When you're relaxed, you breathe approximately fifteen times per minute. That number decreases in deeper states of rest and escalates with increased exercise or nervous tension. In a single day, you inhale approximately 23,000 times, which amounts to transporting about two gallons of air every minute, or 3,000 gallons daily. As the only internal organ to interact with the outside environment, your lungs are vulnerable to dryness and certain weather conditions. So it's always best to protect them from cold and damp weather by keeping your chest, neck, head, and feet warm.

Every function of your body relies for existence on the oxygen intake of the lungs. In fact, each cell performs as a miniature lung by taking in oxygen from the bloodstream and eliminating carbon dioxide, which is then carried back to the lungs. That's why it's so essential for your lungs to have good quality air that is clean, moist, warm, and rich in oxygen. When your lungs aren't functioning properly, your body accumulates heat, propelling other health issues into motion, resulting in poor circulation, night sweats, excessive perspiration, fatigue, and listlessness. Estimates indicate that 92 million of us nationwide (that's more than 1 out of 3) already struggle with at least one of the more common chronic respiratory diseases: sinusitis, allergies, bronchitis, and asthma. According to the American Lung Association, lung disease ranks third in fatal diseases, taking one out of seven lives.

On the front lines protecting your lungs from illness are the sinuses, which are part of the upper sector of the respiratory tract. They serve as the filters for virus, bacteria, dirt and dust, pollen, and other airborne troublemakers. Sensitive to air quality, your sinuses humidify dry air and regulate temperatures so your lungs are shielded from extremes. They can't always function properly, however, because of an influx of environmental irritants (noxious fumes, dust, or chemical particulates);

advanced technology and its subsequent occupational hazards (rubber epoxy, paint resins, dry cleaning chemicals, solvents); allergies; dental problems; extreme temperatures; and the hustle and bustle of everyday life. Amazingly, an estimated 38 million people nationwide are battling sinus disease.

Yet, of all the culprits frustrating the health of your sinuses (as well as the entire respiratory tract), cigarettes and secondhand smoke are among the most insidious. The smoke irritates your mucous membranes and your sinuses, which swell from the inflammation. When your sinuses become infected, you may swallow the mucus that accompanies the infection, which causes gastro and abdominal upsets as well as loose bowels. Similarly, those small airways in your lungs called the bronchi can also become inflamed and blocked by mucus. If your lungs are consistently exposed to irritants, you could develop a chronic condition of bronchitis, which can in turn reduce the oxygen–carbon dioxide process and force your heart to pump harder to make up the slack. Eventually, you could suffer from pulmonary hypertension, an enlarged heart, or complete heart failure.

Since pesticides are used in the growing and processing of tobacco, you are creating a window of opportunity for xenohormones and their byproduct, toxic overload. If you want an image of how your lungs look after such an invasion, take a peek at the brownish residue on a used cigarette filter. (Autumn is an excellent season for letting go of old patterns and opening up to new, healthy ones. What better time to drop your nicotine habit than right now while you're on your journey to better health and *living* beauty?)

But keep in mind that cigarettes aren't the only problem. Smoke from cigars, pipes, campfires, cooking, marijuana, and even cocaine (smoked or snorted) can also damage your mucous membrane. The cold, hard fact is that secondhand smoke is considered even more lethal since it isn't filtered. The sixteen or more known poisons produced by cigarette smoke exist at higher levels than what the smoker actually puffs through the filter! This startling study of nonsmokers—conducted in 1992 by a research group at Harvard—provided the first documented medical evidence that secondhand smoke kills 4,000 annually from lung cancer, increases respiratory infections in children, and aggravates symptoms of asthma.

Reality check: (1) The level of carbon dioxide in people exposed to secondhand smoke is 50 percent higher than in people who aren't invaded by the toxins of a burning cigarette; (2) According to the American Heart Association, secondhand smoke can also be linked to an estimated 40,000 deaths of nonsmokers annually; (3) The American Heart Association also estimates that 50 million adults (nonsmokers over the age of thirty-five) are exposed to the dangers of secondhand smoke and that 50 percent of the children throughout our nation reside in a home where at least one person smokes.

I've stated throughout this book the extreme importance of maintaining a pollutant-free inner and outer environment. Your well-being and beauty are about not just the foods you eat, but also the air you breathe and the things surrounding you. This topic is so critical to the success of your cleansing process that I've dedicated chapter 10 to discussing several ways you can detoxify your outer environment to ensure increased health.

However, an impaired respiratory tract can do even more damage; it can also affect the quality of your skin. Much like a third lung, your skin has cells that breathe and help excrete toxins through perspiration. Both Chinese and Western medical approaches have long linked skin problems to the lungs, particularly eczema, skin rashes, dry, blotchy skin, chapped lips, cracked nails, acne, and psoriasis.

Equally important to your health and detox process are your large intestines, which also need your special attention during autumn. Lying along the outer edge of the abdomen, your large intestine is divided into three parts: the caecum, where your appendix is attached; colons—ascending, transverse, descending, and sigmoid; and the rectum. This five-foot, often-overworked organ absorbs water and finishes nutrient absorption so its blood vessels can transport it to the liver for further metabolism. The main function of your colon is to gather your body's putrefied toxins and eliminate them via peristalsis so the entire system can work without undue stress.

Your gut is like a fortress, maintaining a protective environment where food can be broken down and fed to voracious cells waiting for much-needed nutrients. Its thin mucous membrane absorbs vital nutrients and expels toxins. In a healthy gastrointestinal tract, there are literally trillions of bacteria—good and bad ones. As long as they stay in balance, things are fine. In fact, symbiotes (good intestinal bacteria, like acidophilus and bifidobacteria) help digest and absorb nutrients, make vitamins to defend you from troublesome bacteria, and encourage your immune system.

But when the population of pathogenic bacteria (such as salmonella, staphylococcus, proteus, listeria, campylobacter, clostridium) escalates, a condition called dysbiosis, or leaky gut, occurs. The fortress is ravaged, permitting toxic wastes, bacteria, fungi, undigested proteins, and parasites to enter the bloodstream through its now-porous membrane. Once these substances are in the bloodstream, they can invade your entire body and cause havoc by debilitating your immune system, instigating digestive problems, and taxing the liver. In defense, your body manufactures antibodies, which enter tissues and cause inflammation and arthritic symptoms. In fact, Dr. Jeffrey Bland and his HealthComm International, Inc., in Gig Harbor, Washington, conducted research that showed a connection between an increased number of toxins entering the body through a leaky gut and arthritis, inflammatory joint disease, digestive problems, and below-normal energy levels. He also noted that as we age, our GI tract becomes less efficient, permitting more toxins to escape through the intestinal wall.

And when your system becomes backed up with toxins, a mucus buildup along the lining of the intestinal wall occurs. The wastes lodged in your colon ultimately affect every part of your body and result in constipation. One of the first places this intestinal problem appears is your skin in the form of rashes, blotchy areas, acne, and eczema. And since constipation can cause fecal matter to stay lodged in your system for weeks or even years, this motionless waste develops a hard, stubborn buildup along the walls of the bowels and creates a dangerous playground for unwanted bacteria. It becomes a direct link to various illnesses, such as diverticulitis, ulcer formations, and even degenerative diseases of the digestive tract. Did you know that most of us are carrying around anywhere from seven to ten pounds of encrusted fecal matter in our colons? No wonder we're feeling sluggish! And as this backed-up waste accumulates in our system, it creates a toxic state that can show up as impaired digestion, gas, bloating, headaches, irritability, anxiety, fatigue, mental fog, allergic reactions such as sneezing and watery eyes, and even joint pains and arthritic symptoms. Diets rich in sugar, flour products, and dairy—with their mucus-building properties—as well as alcohol, caffeine, and the Pill can also aggravate your gut. One thing is for certain: disease probably begins in an unhealthy colon.

The Living Beauty Detox Diet for Autumn

Following the detox diet designed for autumn will help you begin to cleanse your system by expelling toxins from the large intestine, thereby helping to prevent autointoxication. Helpful in this regard is the colonic irrigation suggested for the season, which will further purge your system of accumulated wastes and help prevent absorption of new toxins.

Healing Tea, Herbs, and Spices for Autumn

Fenugreek tea is the autumn herbal tea of choice because it is so effective as a lubricant; it softens and dissolves mucus in the lungs and moistens the intestinal tract to prevent constipation. Other lung-protecting herbs include usnea, which the Native Americans fondly named "the Lungs of the Earth," because it works against "bad" bacteria like staphylococcus, streptococcus, pneumonococcus, and mycobacterium tuberculosis; osha, which is a powerful aid for bronchial irritations and has immune-stimulating properties; mullein, which has long been associated with alleviating pulmonary problems because it is an expectorant; and lobelia, a strong bronchial dilator and antispasmodic useful for overall lung congestion and asthma. Autumn spices include warming cinnamon, cloves, nutmeg, and anise, which not only are deliciously aromatic but also help to prevent indigestion, gas, and cold hands and feet. Anise is a lung remedy as well, known to help bronchial disorders and asthma. Your autumn tea, herbs, and spices all help to support intestinal and respiratory function and to alleviate dampness.

Following the Autumn Detox Plan

The harvest season is the time to decrease your intake of cooling summer foods and to add more cooked and warming foods (like velvety okra and crunchy snow peas) into your eating plan in preparation for winter. It is also the season to reduce your fruit intake from three portions to two because fruits are especially cooling to the body. We need more warmth now.

For the autumn detox plan, whether you stay on it for the minimum of three days or for two weeks, the foods to be consumed for breakfast, lunch, and dinner come from the food groups listed below. Sauerkraut from summer, which protects the GI tract, is also included in autumn because we are now working on the lower portion of the GI tract, the large intestine or colon. To further assist in digestive tract cleansing, I suggest a special healing tonic—organic, unfiltered, raw apple cider vinegar—to replace the cooling lemon and lime juices from spring and summer. Organic, unfiltered, raw apple cider vinegar balances the body's pH, provides easily available potassium so helpful to mineral balance and balanced detoxification, and is a natural antiseptic for overall health, including respiratory health. You may use unsalted, natural chicken broth and beef broth for special dishes on the menu plans if you need more liquids for basting or sautéing beyond the limit of 2 tablespoons of oil.

	Autumn Detox Plan Protocol
Oils	1 tablespoon lignan-rich flaxseed oil and 1 tablespoon sesame oil. Sesame oil has a nutty flavor and is high in an antioxidant known as sesamol, which helps to preserve its freshness and stability.
Lean Protein	(at least 8 ounces per day) Beef, buffalo, eggs, lamb, poultry, tofu, and tempeh
Vegetables	Unlimited, raw or steamed, low glycemic. Broccoli, brussels sprouts, cabbage (Chinese cabbage or bok choy), cauliflower, celery, celeriac, celery root, daikon radish,* eggplant, green beans, kale, kohlrabi, lettuce, mushrooms (wild: chanterelle, morel), mustard greens, onions (chives, green, leeks, scallions, shallots), okra, parsley, peppers (green, red, and yellow), radish, snowpeas 3 tablespoons sauerkraut *Daikon, a long white radish, assists digestion and metabolization of fats according to Oriental medicine

	Autumn Detox Plan Protocol, continued
Fruits	1 medium apple (Cortland, Golden Delicious, Gravenstein, Jonathan, or Macintosh); 1 cup cranberries, 1 medium pear, ½ medium persimmon, ½ pomegranate
	1–2 tablespoons apple cider vinegar
Filtered Water	8 glasses a day to rid the body of waste, keep tissues moist, and lubricate the system
With or Between Meals	Take 2 cups of fenugreek tea daily.
Breakfast and Dinner (optional)	Take lung and digestive support supplements containing one or more of the following herbs: lobelia, mullein, osha, and usnea.

Here are some sample days of the Autumn Detox Plan:

	Sample Day One Autumn Detox Plan
Upon Arising	Living Beauty Elixir with 2 high-fiber supplements
	2 eight-ounce glasses of water
Before Breakfast	1 cup fenugreek tea
Breakfast	1 stewed apple with cinnamon and nutmeg
	Autumn Scrambler (made with 2 eggs, mushrooms, and onions with ½ tablespoon sesame seed oil)
Midmorning	2 eight-ounce glasses of water
Lunch	3-ounce tempeh burger
	Warm cabbage salad with grated carrots, celery, and parsley
	Dressing of ½ tablespoon sesame seed oil, 1 tablespoon apple cider vinegar, and ½ teaspoon anise seeds
	3 tablespoons sauerkraut
Midafternoon	2 eight-ounce glasses of water
4 P.M.	1 small pear *Continued*

	Sample Day One Autumn Detox Plan, continued
Dinner	3 ounces broiled lamb chops with dash of cinnamon
	Braised greens and sliced daikon with 1 tablespoon apple cider vinegar and 1 tablespoon flaxseed oil
	Autumn Leaves Veggies (with steamed wild mushrooms, radishes, and snow peas)
	1 cup fenugreek tea
Midevening	Living Beauty Elixir with 2 high-fiber supplements
	2 eight-ounce glasses of water

	Sample Day Two Autumn Detox Plan
Upon Arising	Living Beauty Elixir with 2 high-fiber supplements
	2 eight-ounce glasses of water
Before Breakfast	1 cup fenugreek tea
Breakfast	½ medium sliced baked persimmon
	2 poached eggs
Midmorning	2 eight-ounce glasses of water
Lunch	4-ounce breast of chicken sautéed in 1 tablespoon sesame oil
	Warm cabbage slaw with 1 tablespoon apple cider vinegar
	Steamed green beans
	3 tablespoons sauerkraut
Midafternoon	2 eight-ounce glasses of water
4 P.M.	1 small pear

	Sample Day Two Autumn Detox Plan, continued
Dinner	4 ounces baked scrod with green onions and shallots
	Chopped celeriac, tomato, and scallions with 1 tablespoon flaxseed oil
	1 tablespoon apple cider vinegar
	Roasted eggplant
	1 cup fenugreek tea
Midevening	Living Beauty Elixir with 2 high-fiber supplements
	2 eight-ounce glasses of water

	Sample Day Three Autumn Detox Plan
Upon Arising	Living Beauty Elixir with 2 high-fiber supplements
	2 eight-ounce glasses of water
Before Breakfast	1 cup of fenugreek tea
Breakfast	½ pomegranate
	Tofu Scramble (made with 2 ounces tofu, onions, and chives, topped with 1 tablespoon flaxseed oil)
Midmorning	2 eight-ounce glasses of water
Lunch	Egg salad of 2 hard-boiled eggs, chopped celery, and onion with ½ tablespoon sesame oil and 1 tablespoon apple cider vinegar
	Mixed Autumn Veggies
	3 tablespoons sauerkraut
Midafternoon	2 eight-ounce glasses of water
4 P.M.	1 medium Golden Delicious apple

Continued

	Sample Day Three Autumn Detox Plan, continued
Dinner	4 ounces broiled sea bass
	Warmed daikon with 1 tablespoon apple cider vinegar
	Braised brussels sprouts
	Okra and zucchini sautéed in ½ tablespoon sesame oil
	1 cup fenugreek tea
Midevening	Living Beauty Elixir with 2 high-fiber supplements
	2 eight-ounce glasses of water

Autumn Maintenance Plan

As in the other seasonal detox plans, you can stay on the basic Autumn Detox for as long as two weeks if that is what is indicated from your Living Beauty Cleansing Questionnaire results in chapter 3. Those who would like to increase your menu options and move on to the bountiful maintenance plan can choose from a large variety of fiber-rich harvest vegetables as colorful as the autumn leaves. I would also suggest that you continue taking fenugreek tea and the Living Beauty Elixir with 2 high-fiber supplements at least once a day. Now you may add back foods from the autumn family (vegetables, beans, grains, and breads) beginning with one serving at a time in the portions listed below. The golden autumn grains, quinoa and amaranth, are known as "heirloom" grains and are not only delicate and delicious but hypoallergenic as well. You will also notice spelt on the list as a bagel or bread choice. Spelt is considered a wheat alternative, and although it contains some gluten, most sensitive people are able to tolerate spelt without any difficulty. Luckily, you will have a chance to sample a little bit of everything because, weight permitting, you can ultimately include up to four servings a day from each of the starch families.

You will also note that the dairy selections include not only the lighter yogurts and cottage cheeses from spring and summer but also the heavier, more sustaining, natural, organic cheeses, which can serve as a protein alternative or snack by themselves. I suggest you look for organic goat milk cheeses, which seem to be better tolerated by most people. If you cannot find organic or goat milk cheeses, then to maintain the highest purity standards for your maintenance program, select white cheese over yellow whenever possible because the yellow cheeses are often colored with artificial coloring.

Now is also the time to enjoy more full-bodied, richer foods like nuts and seeds, eating them as snacks or adding them to stir-frys and stews. Enjoy heartier, more sustaining foods that will be warming and help protect you from cooler, and often damper, weather.

The Autumn Starchy Vegetables Selection

One serving of starchy vegetables equals any one of the following:

Acorn squash—½ cup

*Burdock root—½ root

Butternut squash—⅔ cup

Carrots—1 cup

Chestnuts—4 large or 6 small

Corn—½ cup

Green peas—½ cup

†Lotus Root—½ cup

‡Jerusalem artichokes or sunchokes—½ cup

Okra—1 cup

Pumpkin—1 cup

Rutabagas (raw)—¼ large

Sweet potato or yam—½ medium

Turnips—½ cup

* *In Chinese medicine, burdock, a medicinal root vegetable, is well respected for its blood-building and -purifying properties.*

† *According to Chinese medicine, lotus root removes dampness from the lungs.*

‡ *Jerusalem artichokes are high in inulin, the prebiotic, or friendly, undigested carbohydrate that feeds intestinal bacteria.*

The Autumn Beans Selection

One serving of beans equals any one of the following:

Kidney beans—½ cup

Navy (white or great northern)—½ cup

The Autumn Grains and Bread Selection

One serving of grains and bread equals any one of the following:

Quinoa—½ cup

Amaranth—½ cup

Barley—½ cup

Bagel, spelt—½ small

Bread, spelt—1 slice

The Autumn Nuts Selection

One serving of nuts equals any one of the following (except for pumpkinseeds, which are unlimited since high in zinc):

Almonds—½ ounce

Almond butter—2 tablespoons

Cashews—¼ ounce

Cashew butter—1 tablespoon

Filberts or hazelnuts—1 ounce

Macadamia nuts—1 ounce

Peanuts—½ ounce

Peanut butter—1 tablespoon

Pecans—½ ounce

Pine nuts—½ ounce

Pistachio nuts—½ ounce

Pumpkin seeds—unlimited

Sunflower seeds—2 ounces

Sesame seeds—1 ounce

Sesame seed butter—1½ tablespoons

The Autumn Dairy Selection

One serving of dairy equals any one of the following:

Cottage cheese—½ cup

Feta—1 ounce

Gjetost—1 ounce

Goat—1 ounce

Mozzarella (buffalo and cow's milk)—1 ounce

Muenster—1 ounce

Neufchatel—1 ounce

Ricotta, from whole or skim milk—¼ cup

Autumn Maintenance Menu Plan

See the following page for a sample day of the Autumn Maintenance Menu Plan:

	Sample Day Autumn Maintenance Plan
Upon Arising	Living Beauty Elixir with 2 high-fiber supplements
	2 eight-ounce glasses of water
Before Breakfast	1 cup fenugreek tea
Breakfast	½ cup warm applesauce
	½ cup cooked quinoa with ½ tablespoon flaxseed oil
	1 ounce chopped filberts
Midmorning	2 eight-ounce glasses of water
Lunch	4-ounce grilled chicken breast
	Braised brussels sprouts with pearl onions and dash of nutmeg
	1 tablespoon apple cider vinegar
	Autumn Harvest Mixed Green Salad (with seasonally available leafy greens and ½ tablespoon sesame oil)
Midafternoon	2 eight-ounce glasses of water
4 P.M.	1 ounce goat cheese
	1 medium pear
Dinner	4 ounces broiled tempeh burger
	Bok choy sautéed in ½ tablespoon sesame oil
	½ cup acorn squash
	3 tablespoons sauerkraut and 1 teaspoon anise seed
Midevening	2 eight-ounce glasses of water

Autumn Exercises

As the weather turns cooler you must also drink a lot of water because urine output triples in volume when the weather is cold. Water hydrates body tissues and will help keep a stabilized body temperature. Remember to do any warm-up exercises indoors before exercising outdoors; this will acclimate your body to stressful colder temperatures.

Try to get outside as much as you can before winter drives you indoors. As discussed previously, natural sunlight is a key to the cyclical depression syndrome known as Seasonal Affective Disorder (SAD), which occurs in fall when daylight starts to dwindle. Symptoms such as depression, lethargy, and overeating (especially carbohydrates) can begin in October when daylight lessens.

Great autumn exercises include brisk aerobic walking, cycling, jumping rope, and martial arts—especially good for the cardiovascular system. No matter what your age, choose one of the above three days a week for at least thirty minutes each day. When you are exercising outside, even if the weather is still warm, protect your neck with a scarf. According to Traditional Chinese Medicine, the back of the neck is most vulnerable to autumn wind chills. For women in their thirties, forties, fifties, and beyond, strength training at least twice a week for about 45 minutes each time is highly recommended. For those with extremely low bone density, opt for cycling on a stationary bike rather than extreme activities! Stretching and toning on a daily basis is good for all age groups.

Autumn Supporting Treatments for Respiration and Colon

Aromatherapy and Nasal Irrigation

Pollutants such as dust and pollen can bombard the nasal passages every day, inhibiting breathing and irritating the mucous membranes, especially in the autumn. Essential oils from eucalyptus and peppermint as well as a camphorated salve can help clear up nasal passages. Acting as decongestants and stimulants, these oils seem to help circulation to both the nasal and sinus mucous membranes. You can use a drop of eucalyptus oil or peppermint oil on a tissue and simply hold it in front of your nose for a minute or two. You can also put a small drop on your fingertip, spreading the oil around the outside of your nostrils. For more chronic respiratory ailments like bronchitis, asthma, and sinusitis, the camphorated salve can be applied to the chest area two or three times a day.

Seawater rinses are additional helpful breathing aids. They unclog the hair lining the nasal passages, allowing them to effectively filter foreign materials. For more information, see the Resources section.

Colon Therapy

Autumn is the season you may also want to consider a series of colon hydrotherapy treatments to assist in cleansing the bowel. This involves irrigating the entire length of the colon or large intestines with a lukewarm solution. The solution dislodges and removes toxins from hard-to-reach pockets where fecal matter has a tendency to accumulate, impact, and putrefy. The procedure takes about three-quarters of an hour and is usually conducted in a health professional's office by a certified colon hydrotherapist. Make sure your colon therapist uses water that has been filtered to remove chemicals, heavy metals, and parasites. You may also want to be assured that additional antiseptic measures such as the use of disposable tubing are part of the procedure.

Colon hydrotherapists believe (and I can attest to this as a regular colonic devotee for over twenty years) regular colon cleansing helps relieve a number of stubborn skin problems as well as dark circles and bags under the eyes. Skin texture, hydration, color, and clarity all improve, and fatigue, gas, headaches, and irritability are lessened. Colonic enthusiasts report a marked sense of well-being, more energy, less brain fog, and more tranquillity. Colon hydrotherapy can help establish the pattern of regular bowel movements on a daily basis. Once the system has been cleansed with colon hydrotherapy, the colon can again function as it was meant to, eliminating unwanted wastes from the body.

7

Winter Seasonal Detox Diet

A winter scene is awe-inspiring in its beauty and silence.
SUZANNE CAYGILL,
founder of the four-season color-harmony theory

The winter solstice, occurring on December 21, whispers the beginning of winter. The beauty of its stillness envelops you. You're quieted and begin to ponder inward reflections. Since the days are much shorter, you're aware of the need to get more natural sunlight to ward off effects of SAD, the Seasonal Affective Disorder caused by light deprivation. And you take special care to nurture the organs of the season, the kidneys and adrenal glands.

Your kidneys and bladder work harmoniously in the detox process to eliminate wastes from your system. The kidneys filter blood to a balance between water and the body's acidity level. They help your system keep the right amounts of sodium, potassium, chlorine, calcium, magnesium, and phosphate while helping to pull out elements like nitrogen, minerals, salts, and unwanted chemicals. In one day, the kidney filters several thousand quarts of blood, of which approximately 160 quarts of fluid are extracted for another filtering process. When the filtering is complete, only one or two quarts are left to eliminate. Urine flows from the kidneys to the urethras, then to the bladder—a muscular organ located in the pelvis— where it is eliminated. The kidneys and bladder as well as the skin excrete water from the body: urine from the kidneys and bladder and sweat from the skin. In fact, urine and perspiration share similar chemistry.

When your kidneys become weakened, their lack of energy ripples throughout your body. Your skin is forced to do double time in the elimi- nation process, which causes rashes and other skin conditions to appear. Your liver and lung as well as ovary functions become impaired, giving rise to menopauselike symptoms: hot flashes, night sweats, irritability, insomnia, sleep problems, pains in joints, and breast tenderness.

And if your liver becomes burdened with too many toxins, the excess passes into the bloodstream and infiltrates your kidneys, which are not equipped to detoxify the wastes. Consequently, the toxic substances move on to the urinary tract or outward through your skin. Irritated by these poisons, your urinary tract is a doormat for yeast infections, viruses, and bacteria.

That's why it's important to check the color, clarity, and tone of your skin. A kidney problem may cause a bluish discoloration around the eyes. Also look at your hair. If it is too oily, too dry, thinning, or too thick, it may indicate an imbalance in the kidneys and bladder.

Stress, whether it's environmental, emotional, or physical, places a great hardship on your adrenal glands. Situated on top of your kidneys, your adrenals (stress glands) are on the alert every second of the day, responding to the pressures affecting you. In order to cope, the adrenals manufacture hormones such as adrenaline and cortisol, a steroid known as the stress hormone. Cortisol is an extremely important adrenal hor- mone because it keeps blood sugar levels in check so every cell in your body receives the energy it needs to keep you going, no matter what stressful situation is occurring—an infection, a heat wave, or a hot flash. The more your adrenals are under siege because of unrelenting physical, emotional, or psychological stress, the greater the likelihood of burnout or adrenal exhaustion

Sluggish adrenals are a hallmark of zinc deficiency and copper overload. Whenever your adrenal functions are decreased, they can no longer signal the liver to detoxify and excrete excess copper through their protein carrier escort known as ceruloplasmin. Depressed adrenal function can create various secondary symptoms such as chronic fatigue or exhaustion; low blood pressure; food or environmental allergies; low immune function; hypoglycemia or diabetes; PMS or menopause difficulties (such as hot flashes, irritability, weight gain); an inability to handle stress; salt cravings (because of low sodium levels); or cravings for sweets (to give you quick energy).

However, adrenal stress can provoke other health concerns. Your eyes may become too sensitive to light because your pupil contractions have slowed, forcing you to don sunglasses much of the time. You also might feel dizzy if you get up too soon because of a sudden drop in blood pressure.

Another major concern during the winter season is the decrease in daylight, which I talked about in the previous chapter. Winter puts you at greater risk for SAD, the Seasonal Affective Disorder. Many women, especially under the age of forty-five, seem to be sensitive to light deprivation and end up battling depression. They turn inward, become more isolated and lethargic, and even seem to be more susceptible to illnesses. And some symptoms of SAD can mimic other conditions, from chronic fatigue and PMS to hypoglycemia and hypothyroidism.

You can't underestimate the importance of sunlight, which is a nutrient having a catalytic effect on your body's glands. Although there is not a known cure for SAD, studies have shown that over half of the study participants improved by getting concentrated doses of bright light each morning. Keeping blinds or curtains open to expose more of the daylight throughout the day is one approach. However, you may also want to invest in full-spectrum light bulbs, which have also been known to help and are now available in natural food stores and natural markets.

The Living Beauty Detox Diet for Winter

Following the detox diet designed for winter will help you begin to cleanse your system by expelling toxins from the kidneys, the primary organs of detoxification. Replenishing your entire system at this time of the year through adequate rest, relaxation, and meditation is key to regenerating and renewing your kidneys—as well as your stress glands, the adrenals.

Healing Tea, Herbs, and Spices for Winter

Nettle tea is the wintertime herbal tea of choice because it is a rich source of alkalizing minerals especially helpful for kidney cleansing and adrenal support. Other kidney-protecting herbs include juniper berries, which act as a diuretic and are especially helpful in chronic bladder infections; gingerroot, which is warming to the body and helps circulation in the kidney area; and marshmallow root, which is good for soothing mucous membrane irritation in the urinary tract. The natural sodium and other electrolytes in unrefined sea salt and miso assist both kidney and adrenal functions. Miso is a fermented soybean product that is especially noteworthy because it also strengthens the blood and lymph and is a good source of enzymes, calcium, and iron. Tamari, an aged soy sauce, is a flavorful alternative to salt and aids digestion. Ginger can also be used as a seasoning in cooking.

Following the Winter Detox Plan

During this season of stillness and rest, your foods for detox should be cooked or warmed so your body's energy is freed to sustain body heat and immunity. Your water, especially, at this time of year should not be iced or cold, which shocks the system, but should be taken at room temperature. For the winter detox plan, whether you are on it for three days or two weeks based on your responses to the Living Beauty Cleansing Questionnaire in chapter 3, the foods to be consumed for breakfast, lunch, and dinner should be chosen from the food groups listed below. Both sauerkraut and apple cider vinegar are included in winter's detox plan. You will note that this season is the only time when natural salt and tamari are purposefully allowed. Miso is a valuable winter seasoning because it provides some immune-boosting benefits as well as a natural salt that supports the kidneys and adrenals. As with the other detoxification programs, you may use unsalted chicken broth and beef broth for special dishes on the menu plans if you need more liquids for basting or sautéing beyond the limit of 2 tablespoons of oil.

	Winter Detox Plan Protocol
Oil	Choose 1 tablespoon of lignan-rich flaxseed oil and 1 tablespoon of sesame oil, which is tasty as well as high in a natural antioxidant known as sesamol, resistant to oxidation.
Lean Protein	(at least 8 ounces per day) Choose beef, buffalo, deer, eggs, elk, fish, seafood. and poultry.
Vegetables	Unlimited, raw or steamed, low glycemic. Choose broccoli, brussels sprouts, cabbage (red, green, Chinese, or bok choy), cauliflower, celery, celeriac, daikon radish, eggplant, green beans, lettuce, mushrooms (boletu, chanterelle, morel, shiitake), mustard greens, onions (chives, green, leeks, scallions, and shallots), parsley, peppers (green, red, and yellow), radish, snow peas.
Fruits	Apples (Cortland, Jonathan, Macintosh, Pippin, Rome Beauty), applesauce (unsweetened, organic, ½ cup), apple-cranberry sauce (unsweetened, organic, ½ cup), 1 cup cranberries, 1 small pear (d'Anjou), 1 tangerine
Filtered Water	8 glasses a day to rid the body of waste, keep tissues moist, and lubricate the system
With or Between Meals	Take 1 cup of nettle tea daily.
Breakfast and Dinner (optional)	Take a kidney/adrenal support supplement containing 1 or more of the following herbs: juniper berries, gingerroot, horsetail, and marshmallow root.

Here are some sample days of the Winter Detox Plan:

	Day One Winter Detox Plan
Upon Arising	Living Beauty Elixir with 2 high-fiber supplements
	2 eight-ounce glasses of water
Before Breakfast	1 cup nettle tea *Continued*

	Day One Winter Detox Plan, continued
Breakfast	½ cup apple-cranberry sauce
	2 ounces breakfast steak with sautéed shiitake mushrooms, onions, and celery in 1 tablespoon sesame oil
Midmorning	2 eight-ounce glasses of water
Lunch	3 ounces broiled buffalo burger
	Wilted winter salad of cabbage, daikon, and celery with 1 tablespoon flaxseed oil and 1 tablespoon apple cider vinegar
	Braised string beans and zucchini with ¼ teaspoon salt
Midafternoon	2 eight-ounce glasses of water
4 P.M.	1 Rome Beauty apple
Dinner	Stuffed peppers, made with 3 ounces ground turkey, daikon, and celery with ⅛ teaspoon tamari
	Braised mustard greens and onions
	Grilled winter mushrooms
	3 tablespoons sauerkraut
	1 cup nettle tea
Midevening	Living Beauty Elixir with 2 high-fiber supplements
	2 eight-ounce glasses of water

	Sample Day Two Winter Detox Plan
Upon Arising	Living Beauty Elixir with 2 high-fiber supplements
	2 eight-ounce glasses of water
Before Breakfast	1 cup nettle tea
Breakfast	2 ounces tempeh burger with ⅛ teaspoon miso
	½ cup applesauce
Midmorning	2 eight-ounce glasses of water

	Sample Day Two Winter Detox Plan, continued
Lunch	3-ounce hamburger with sliced onions, mushrooms, and parsley
	Baked cauliflower finished with 1 tablespoon flaxseed oil
	3 tablespoons sauerkraut
Midafternoon	2 eight-ounce glasses of water
4 P.M.	1 tangerine
Dinner	4 ounces sea bass broiled with 1 tablespoon sesame oil, ¼ teaspoon tamari, and ¼ teaspoon grated ginger
	Grated daikon, carrot, and onion salad drizzled with 1 tablespoon apple cider vinegar
	Medley of steamed broccoli, cauliflower, and snow peas
	1 cup nettle tea
Midevening	Living Beauty Elixir with 2 high-fiber supplements
	2 eight-ounce glasses of water

	Sample Day Three Winter Detox Plan
Upon Arising	Living Beauty Elixir with 2 high-fiber supplements
	2 eight-ounce glasses of water
Before Breakfast	1 cup nettle tea
Breakfast	Baked d'Anjou pear
	2 scrambled eggs with diced onions, parsley, and a dash of salt
Midmorning	2 eight-ounce glasses of water
Lunch	3 ounces broiled chicken cutlet with ¼ teaspoon tamari
	Grilled eggplant and tomato garnish finished with 1 tablespoon apple cider vinegar
	1 tablespoon flaxseed oil

Continued

	Sample Day Three Winter Detox Plan, continued
Midafternoon	2 eight-ounce glasses of water
4 P.M.	1 baked apple
Dinner	3 ounces shrimp with red and green cabbage and carrots sautéed in 1 tablespoon sesame oil
	Snow peas
	3 tablespoons sauerkraut
	1 cup nettle tea
Midevening	Living Beauty Elixir with 2 high-fiber supplements
	2 eight-ounce glasses of water

Winter Maintenance Plan

You can maintain the basic winter detox menu for up to two weeks if the Living Beauty Cleansing Questionnaire results from chapter 3 indicate that you need a longer cleanse. But those of you who are ready for maintenance may make a number of warming additions to the basic Winter Detox Plan that will sustain your cleansing momentum while nourishing and supporting you during the cold. I do suggest that you continue with winter's nettle tea and the Living Beauty Elixir with 2 high-fiber supplements at least once a day.

Now you may add back food from the starch family (vegetables, beans, grains, or breads), beginning with one serving at a time. Warming, fiber-rich kasha and whole-grain rye, so beneficial for revving up circulation, can be enjoyed in the cold of winter. So can sprouted bagels and breads and whole-grain rye bread. You can ultimately include up to four servings a day from each of the starch selections.

Also, you may include cheese as a snack or protein substitute, and you get a special treat—nuts and seeds for crunchy wintertime snacks or as additions to your wintry stir-frys, salads, or stews. For greater variety you will also now have the option of nitrate-free turkey or chicken sausage as well as nitrate-free turkey bacon.

The Winter Starchy Vegetables Selection

One serving of vegetables equals any one of the following:

Burdock—½ root

Acorn squash—½ cup

Carrots—1 cup

Chestnuts—4 large or 6 small

Butternut squash—⅔ cup

Jerusalem artichoke or sunchokes—½ cup

Parsnips—⅔ cup

Sweet potato or yam—½ medium

Turnips—½ cup

The Winter Beans Selection

One serving of beans equals any one of the following:

Aduki—½ cup

Black—½ cup

Pinto beans—½ cup

The Winter Grains and Breads

One serving of grains and breads equals any one of the following:

Buckwheat groats or kasha—½ cup

Rye—½ cup

Bagel, sprouted grain—½ bagel

Bread, rye—1 slice

Bread, sprouted—1 slice

The Winter Dairy Selection

One serving of dairy equals any one of the following:

Cottage cheese—½ cup

Feta—1 ounce

Gjetost—1 ounce

Goat—1 ounce

Beef sausage—1 ounce

Chicken sausage—1 ounce

Turkey sausage—1 ounce

Winter Nuts Selection

One serving of nuts equals any one of the following (except pumpkin seeds, which are unlimited because they are high in zinc):

Almonds—½ ounce

Almond butter—2 tablespoons

Cashews—½ ounce

Cashew butter—1 tablespoon

Coconut milk—¼ cup

Coconut meat—¼ shredded

Filberts or hazelnuts—1 ounce

Macadamia nuts—1 ounce

Peanuts—½ ounce

Peanut butter—1 tablespoon

Pecans—½ ounce

Pine nuts—½ ounce

Pistachio nuts—½ ounce

Pumpkin seeds—unlimited

Sunflower seeds—1 ounce

Sesame seeds—½ ounce

Sesame seed butter—1 tablespoon

Winter Maintenance Menu Plan

Here is a sample day of the Winter Maintenance Menu Plan:

	Sample Day Winter Maintenance Plan
Upon Arising	Living Beauty Elixir with 2 high-fiber supplements
	2 eight-ounce glasses of water
Before Breakfast	1 cup nettle tea
Breakfast	½ cup apple-cranberry sauce
	2 ounces organic turkey sausage or 2 ounces of turkey
	½ sprouted bagel and ½ tablespoon flaxseed oil
Midmorning	2 eight-ounce glasses of water
Lunch	3 ounces roasted turkey
	Braised spinach and red cabbage with 1 tablespoon apple cider vinegar
	⅔ cup butternut squash with ½ tablespoon flaxseed oil
Midafternoon	2 eight-ounce glasses of water
4 P.M.	1 tangerine
Dinner	3 ounces beef patty
	Celery root salad with 1 tablespoon apple cider vinegar
	Steamed Winter Vegetable Potpourri with 1 tablespoon sesame oil and ½ teaspoon tamari
Midevening	2 eight-ounce glasses of water

Winter Exercises

In cold weather, clothing should be loose rather than tight fitting. Choose the layered look, consisting of several layers of natural material. Insulation is provided through the warm, air-filled spaces between the layers. Plastic fabrics or polyester should be avoided because these fabrics do not allow the skin to breathe (and plastic is a xenohormonic substance). Do remember to keep your head and neck covered to protect body heat from escaping. Also try to stay dry. Melting snow and rain create moisture, affecting clothing insulation. Water removes body heat at least twenty times faster than air.

For those of you who are in your teens, twenties, thirties, and forties, winter sports that are good for cardiovascular health include downhill skiing, cross-country skiing, snowshoeing, and shoveling snow. Try to enjoy these at least three times a week for thirty minutes. If the weather outside is frightful, then some great indoor winter cardiovascular exercises like jumping rope or working out to a cardiovascular exercise video can be alternated. For women in their thirties, forties, fifties, and beyond, twice-a-week strength training for about forty-five minutes builds strong bones and helps to burn fat during the more sedentary wintertime. Other indoor sports like martial arts, yoga, and tai chi as well as stretching and toning exercises can be enjoyed by every age group. Try to do these at least three times a week for about twenty to thirty minutes each time. When it comes to winter sports, let moderation be your guide. Don't overdo it and burn out your energy reserves, which you should be replenishing at this time.

Wintertime Supporting Treatments During Detox and Beyond

Since winter is the time for cleansing and supporting the kidneys and the adrenals, both rest and relaxation techniques are healing and rejuvenating. The following are my top suggestions for lessening stress and improving both kidney and adrenal function.

Develop good sleeping habits (try to be in bed by 10 P.M.) and take some time each day for rest and relaxation. Take frequent breaks from stress by doing whatever works best to lighten your stress load, whether that is reading comic books, listening to music, stretching, or doing deep breathing, meditating, or affirmations. (Please refer to chapter 9, "Detoxing the Inner," for more specific guidance.)

Set priorities and stick with them. Save your energy for things that are important or are rewarding to you. Fill your life with as many things as possible that give you pleasure and promote positive feelings.

Break the worry habit. Continually remind yourself that worrying won't change what is happening in your life, but the distress you feel from it will take its toll on your body's ability to overcome exhaustion.

Take control of your life and your time, and don't blame others for your problems. Instead, learn to express yourself and tell people close to you what you really want and need from them. Make it a point not to take on responsibilities you'd rather not do (and will later resent).

Do light-to-moderate wintertime exercise, because physical activity typically lessens stress, but it is important not to push yourself so far that you further deplete adrenal energy. Exercise at the level that feels best to you, even if that is only a short yoga stretch.

Simplify your life. Remind yourself that your energy is needed right now to help your body heal from fatigue. Cut back on social activities and obligations that create stress and rob you of energy.

8

Beauty Routines for Ages and Stages

Nature gives you the face you have at twenty;
it's up to you to make the face you have at fifty.
COCO CHANEL

Seasonal cleansing and specific beautifying nutrients are the keys to radiant good looks and glowing health. But let's take a look at the deeper factors, both internal and external, that will maximize your beauty through every age and stage of your life.

Simply stated, many of the beauty problems you may be facing are not necessarily tied to the stage of life you're in. Acne and oily skin are no longer teen problems. Now, thanks to toxic overload, modern-day stress, and the hormone havoc caused by estrogen dominance, these troublesome skin conditions can plague women in their thirties or even forties. All of us, regardless of age, must combat many factors that greatly affect the quality of our beauty—from the sun, climate, and seasons to emotions, hormones, and mineral deficiencies like copper-zinc imbalances.

Copper-zinc imbalances, I can attest, will affect your system at any age. For most of my life, I've had to deal with sensitive skin. It's one of the reasons I became so interested in nutrition in the first place. During college, I battled embarrassing acne. The blemishes seemed to take forever to heal and often left a little reddish mark. I was terrified I'd be scarred for life. I knew only too well how sugary foods, chocolate, nuts, wheat germ, shellfish, and even too much fruit juice could cause my skin to react negatively. Then in the late 1980s, my hair started to develop a strange-looking orange tint. At that same time, I began to feel tired and yet my mind was in overdrive. Many nights were filled with restless sleep. In time, I got to the bottom of my longtime skin problems and the other bizarre symptoms—copper overload and a zinc deficiency. I discovered a variety of supplements as well as natural remedies to help me overcome these health and beauty problems.

As mentioned in chapter 2, excess estrogen or estrogen dominance goes hand in hand with copper retention and deficiencies in zinc and progesterone. Copper overload can further escalate PMS, perimenopausal, and some menopausal symptoms by increasing anxiety, panic attacks, roller-coaster emotions, insomnia, and the syndrome of racing mind accompanying an exhausted body. By displacing zinc, copper depresses adrenal gland function, manifesting on the skin as tanning or dark freckles. Copper destroys vitamin C and the bioflavonoids, thereby weakening collagen and the skin proteins, keratin and elastin.

Although I've categorized the beauty tips in this chapter according to typical age groups, I encourage you to also read the tips and routines that apply to your specific problem, not just your stage of life. Also, please note that some of the seasonal detox maintenance components reappear in this next section because they are an intricate part of the fundamentals of beauty.

The Basic Truths About Beauty:
What Every Body Needs Regardless of Age

Beauty Basic Truth #1: The Sun

First and foremost, I want to modify the skin care law "The sun is your skin's number one enemy." I know you've heard it your whole life, but to be more accurate it should go like this: "The sun is your skin's number one enemy—except for fifteen minutes, three times per week, before 10 A.M. and after 3 P.M." As you have already read, vitamin D, the sunshine vitamin, is critical for developing bones and for absorbing and using calcium—and, subsequently, for preventing osteoporosis. And since sunscreens absorb the UV rays needed for your body to synthesize vitamin D, constant sunscreen use has been found to decrease vitamin D levels in the blood.

You might be thinking, "Wouldn't it be easier to take a vitamin D supplement?" Well, you could, but the form of vitamin D obtained from supplements or foods (like butter, dairy products, eggs, and fish) is not an active form. Besides, the synthetic vitamin D (found in fortified milk) has been shown to impair magnesium absorption in the body. If you take a vitamin D supplement, your liver has to convert it to the active form. And that can be a problem, especially if your liver is heavily taxed already, which is probably the case because it is having to neutralize all the petrochemical pesticides, alcohol, and toxic byproducts of normal digestion and cellular metabolism.

However, sunscreens do have their place. If you're in your teens or twenties, you should take special care and wear sunscreens (at least an SPF 15) that protect against both the sunburning UVB rays as well as the skin cancer–linked UVA rays. Getting both UVB and UVA protection is also particularly necessary among those aged twenty-five to twenty-nine, because skin cancer occurrences in that age group outrank breast cancer, AIDS, and fatal accidents combined! And wearing sunscreen during prime sun time (from 10 A.M. to 3 P.M.) and protecting your lips with a lip balm formulated with sunscreen are equally important for individuals of all ages.

But what kind of sunscreen you choose is critical. Progressive

Canadian researcher and chemist Hans Larsen believes that chemical sunscreens may actually help promote the formation of skin cancer. Larsen has explained that most chemical sunscreens contain benzophenone or its derivatives (oxybenzone, benzophenone-3) as their active ingredients. In an article published in the *International Journal of Alternative and Complementary Medicine,* Larsen wrote, "Benzophenone is one of the most powerful free radical generators known to man." As a safer alternative to sunscreens containing benzophenone, Larsen recommends using sunscreens that contain both titanium dioxide and zinc oxide. He further stated that chemical sunscreens such as benzophenone work by absorbing UVB rays. Inert minerals such as titanium dioxide and zinc oxide, on the other hand, work by reflecting UVA and UVB rays away from the skin instead of absorbing them. This difference makes physical sunscreens much safer to use than chemical ones, according to Larsen. Furthermore, Drs. Cedrick and Frank Garland of the University of California feel certain the increased use of chemical sunscreens is the main cause of the skin cancer epidemic based on these factors:

- Chemical sunscreens absorb UVB radiation but allow most of the deep, penetrating UVA light through. UVA light is involved in the formation of melanoma, one of the fastest-growing cancers if untreated.

- People using sunscreens typically stay in the sun longer, developing a false sense of security. Subsequently, they subject themselves to more damaging UVA rays.

- UVA light, not absorbed by chemical sunscreens, suppresses the immune system. Specifically, it causes a loss of Langerhan's cells, which are immune cells designed to keep the skin healthy and protected from free radical damage, bacteria, and other pathogens.

- Sunscreens protect against sunburn but haven't been proven to protect against melanoma or basal cell carcinoma (another form of skin cancer).

- The greatest rise in melanoma has occurred in countries where chemical sunscreens have been heavily promoted.

- Recent studies conducted by the Garlands demonstrated an increase rate of basal cell carcinoma among women who use sunscreen.

You can naturally boost your skin's SPF if you take certain nutrients internally, according to the research of Dr. Howard Murad of Los Angeles, California: "We recently did a study that found that taking vitamin E, grapeseed extract, antioxidants, and other nutrients that help repair sun damage orally, can actually raise your skin's SPF by 10%." Other experts agree, stating that in addition to using a physical sunscreen to reflect sunlight away from the skin, many studies have suggested that increasing your intake of antioxidants is an important strategy for preventing skin cancer and the damage caused by sun exposure. If you're interested in bumping up your SPF, try supplements containing vitamin A, beta-carotene, vitamin C, vitamin E, selenium, zinc, pine bark, or grapeseed extract. However, the sun is nothing to fool with, so make sure to also wear a protective sunscreen.

Beauty Basic Truth #2: Essential Fatty Acids

As suggested in the seasonal detox maintenance programs, every adult woman should consider taking a daily dose of essential fatty acids (EFAs) in the form of either flaxseed oil or a combination of flaxseed and primrose oils. Both of these oils help greatly in controlling hormonal symptoms related to your menstrual cycle, such as migraine headaches, cramps, and hot flashes. They also have the ability to mobilize calcium—with its desirable qualities of strength and resilience—into the skin, where they contribute to a harder protective surface. Think of it this way: the ozone layer acts as the Earth's protective skin against the sun's harmful rays. Likewise, you need to build up your skin to offset the assault of those harmful rays. And the tougher protection you need is found in EFAs.

Beauty Basic Truth #3: Wrinkle Busters

We can blame the sun for most skin damage, but the truth is that lines and wrinkles can also result from many other factors. Consider some of these top wrinkle promoters:

- Repeated facial expressions: like pouting, frowning, squinting, or pursing your lips.

- Smoking: with each puff, you're curling your lips; that add up to hundreds of times per day. After years of cigarette inhaling, those minor cigarette creases can soon develop into full-fledged wrinkles.

- Alcohol and caffeine: both are diuretics, which tend to make the body lose moisture and consequently dry out the skin, encouraging wrinkles.

- Drugs like cortisone, cortisporin, aspirin, and bronkolixir: can rob you of nutrients like vitamin B_6, zinc, potassium, wrinkle-fighting vitamin C, vitamin D, and vitamin K—all necessary for skin elasticity, tone, and hydration.

- Poor dental work: can make your mouth look skewed, marring your overall appearance.

- A low-protein and fat-free diet: lacks tissue-strengthening protein and the internal moisturizing benefits of the EFAs.

- Lack of exercise: it prevents the system from taking in enough oxygen to oxygenate the tissues for a rosy, glowing complexion.

- Hereditary factors: fair, drier complexions are said to age sooner than darker, oilier skin.

- Environmental stress: from the sun's ultraviolet light and pollutants like cigarette smoke, car exhaust, byproducts of normal metabolism, and all-pervading xenoestrogens. They create free radicals—those unstable molecules of oxygen associated with aging and degenerative disease—which are at the very core of skin damage.

Free Radicals, Antiaging Antioxidants, and Your Skin

And speaking of those nasty free radicals, did you know they can also damage your cell membranes and DNA structure? Just as fabric that sits under the sun for a long time bleaches out and gets weakened fibers, your skin will respond in much the same way. Each fragile cell will in time lose its firmness and begin to sag, causing wrinkles to form. Once the skin's DNA cellular structure is injured, this inferior model is reproduced, creating a deterioration of tissue in every area of the body, including the skin's proteins, collagen, and elastin. Your body can help fight off these unstable molecules to some degree by producing internal free radical scavengers that quench the free radicals before they do damage. And although certain foods—such as antioxidants vitamin C and vitamin E as well as beta-carotene—can also contribute to the fight against free radicals, there are just too many xenoestrogenic substances as well as other pollutants, toxins, heavy metals, chemicals, parasites, and stress these days for your poor liver to contend with. This is why dietary antioxidant supplements have been promoted so heavily in the health food industry.

Of course, antioxidants are also big business in the cosmetic world. When applied as a topical application, these aging-busting antioxidants (especially beauty-enriched vitamins C, E, and A) act like guided missiles, targeting your face, nails, and hair. Internal supplements, on the other hand, may need to be used elsewhere before they make their way to your outer body. This may explain why people who ingest antioxidants don't always have rich vitamin reserves in their skin. Plus, as we get older the body doesn't efficiently deliver vitamins and minerals from the intestinal tract to the outside skin, the last place to receive nutrients. This discovery is profound because it means that the right topical antioxidants can prevent aging.

Although these topical antioxidants seem promising, I've come to the conclusion that there are many problems associated with the topical application of vitamins in cosmetic products. First of all, they may not contain the amount of the vitamin used in clinical studies; second, companies may not be able to stabilize the vitamin adequately enough to prevent degradation. For example, an enormous amount of vitamin C topicals are on the market these days. But how would you, the consumer, know to select products with at least 5 percent to 15 percent vitamin C content in accordance with the amounts used in the clinical studies? How would you know if the product you selected was stable and kept in a cool dark place, since vitamin C is known to break down rapidly? Chances are, you probably wouldn't. In the Resources section you will find names of products that contain the correct amount and type of vitamin C.

Certainly the best researched of the topical antioxidant creams are Retin-A and Renova, which are relatives of vitamin A itself. Although these products are known to smooth skin, reduce fine lines, and even fade age spots, based on scientific studies, they're available only by prescription and can be highly irritating as well as uncomfortable because of the itching and flaking they produce. Retinol, the over-the-counter cousin of vitamin A, is contained in many cosmetic lines; it seems to be a bit kinder to sensitive skin but can be irritating as well.

Lycopene, an antioxidant that appears to reduce the risk of prostate cancer, may very well be the antioxidant of choice. It's a red carotenoid found in tomatoes, pink grapefruit, and watermelon that helps protect you from both UVA and UVB rays. You may want to look for products containing this new promising star.

Or you can save your money and avoid the potential irritation by making your own topical antioxidant skin care treatments. Just open a capsule of vitamin A (25,000 IU) and vitamin E (400 IU), then mix them into your moisturizer. You might want to try this favorite of my clients: crack open a capsule of a high-potency antioxidant that contains vitamins A, C, E, selenium, and zinc and mix it into your day cream and sunscreen for extra antioxidant protection.

You can also save a lot of money by making your own alpha-hydroxies—those new darlings of the cosmetic industry. Alpha-hydroxies break down the cellular mortar that bind cells to one another so that the dead ones can be shed, leaving your skin shiny and new. Many of the most commonly used hydroxies in cosmetics today, however, are contained naturally in sources like sugar cane (glycolic acid), sour milk and yogurt (lactic acid), grapes, papaya, avocado, citrus (fruit acids), honey, and lemon juice. You'll find a number of these kitchen cosmetics in my Natural Tips and Beauty Routines section, which follows. The natural alpha-hydroxies are simple, safe, and effective as well as less stinging and irritating than the commercial versions.

Antiaging Creams

Selecting the best skin care products is confusing, to say the least. Clearly, some of the new topical antioxidant creams not only promise but deliver results because they have the ability to neutralize free radical damage from the sun, which is the worst offender in aging skin. But what about creams that contain collagen, elastin, ginseng, gingko biloba, aloe, chamomile, pregnenolone, emu oil, or RNA and DNA?

Unfortunately, the majority of these products cannot live up to their inflated Madison Avenue marketing claims, according to beauty expert Paula Begoun. Why not? Because of the nature of the aging process itself. The more years under the proverbial belt, the more our skin grows, even though bottom layers are shrinking. Since our bones also decrease with the onslaught of time, and since we lack sufficient muscle or fat to pull the skin up, it droops. Even our facial muscles weaken and lose elasticity. No matter what beauty items we buy or how long and hard we exercise, we can't hold back the ticking of the biological clock. Constant use and damage from the sun also cause the muscles in our face to eventually sag. A plastic surgeon tries to turn back the hands of time by pulling the sagging facial muscles back to their original position. And, as previously mentioned, facial expressions like frowns or furrowed brows also contribute to those unattractive vertical or horizontal facial lines. Since lotions can't stop you from making your facial frowns, furrows, or grimaces, some women resort to injections that erase wrinkles by paralyzing muscles in the forehead.

Growing older also means that collagen and elastin, both vital skin proteins, diminish. Collagen fibers provide the skin's firmness by creating a protein net; elastin fibers give it elasticity. The decrease in these key proteins further reduces the plumping or moisturizing agent. Consequently, the collagen fibers become flaccid and fibrous, and the now-thinning epidermis goes limp, which results in wrinkles and lines. Eventually collagen fibers harden, the elastic tissue decreases, and sagging, wrinkled skin is produced. Since skin is no longer pliant enough to absorb things, a topical beauty product touting its ability to increase collagen or even elastin won't help.

Some other useful substances also diminish with time, such as the hydrating and texture-fortifying elements of hyaluronic acids, ceramides, polysaccharides, enzymes, coenzymes, and proteins. And the autoimmune system may also deteriorate, since aging skin is more conducive to skin sensitivities and even allergies.

At the molecular level, Old Father Time as well as the sun can cause the DNA codes (the principle of the aging process) in skin cells to scramble or get lost. Not only does this retard cell reproduction, it also distorts their shape, which in turn alters the texture of skin and its ability to retain water. This is why our skin becomes drier as we age. Some cosmetic companies try to sell the idea that they can correct this problem by formulating their products with DNA and RNA. But that doesn't work. Besides, playing around with genetic coding isn't smart business. You might even be opening the doorway to cancer.

We're all concerned about aging, so more and more products appear on the market claiming to undo the inevitable. You'll find ceramides, hyaluronic acid, proteins, and types of seaweeds harvested in exotic locations throughout the world listed as ingredients in wrinkle creams. However, neither ceramides or hyaluronic acid—both strong water-drawing agents and somewhat helpful as moisturizers—can be placed back into the skin, either topically or internally, because of their large molecular structure. Even if the substances were altered chemically to permeate the skin, we wouldn't know the correct amount to use. Plus, the actual number of elements your skin is losing is in the thousands. The message? Save your hard-earned money.

Avoiding beauty-robbing petrochemicals (xenoestrogen) as much as possible is paramount, which means no artificial colors, synthetic fragrances, petrolatum or mineral oil, emulsifiers, and solvents in our cleansers, toners, serums, beauty boosters, eye creams, day creams, night creams, facial masks, and moisturizers. This will make choosing body care products much easier for you, since it knocks out about three-fourths of those on the market today, unless of course you shop almost exclusively at health food stores or fine boutiques.

Beauty Basic Truth #4: The Acid Mantle

Just as the atmosphere has a protective mantle known as the ozone layer, your skin has a protective shield known as the acid mantle. It amazes me that nobody talks about the importance of protecting the natural acid mantle of your skin with proper pH-balanced products that match your skin's acid mantle. The pH value is a way of expressing acidity and alkalinity on a scale from 0 to 14. Your skin has a value between 4 and 6, generally taken as 5.5.

So here's one thing I would like you to do, particularly if you have signs of an alkaline pH such as dry or itchy skin or scalp, or dandruff. Start testing all of your cosmetics, hair, and skin care products. All you do is apply a bit of the product (cream, lotion, or serum) to a small strip of nitrazene, or litmus paper, available at drugstores and pharmacies. If the paper turns yellow, the product is on the acidic side, which is what you want. However, if the paper turns blue or purplish, the product is alkaline, which is what you don't want. Your goal is to match your skin's natural acid mantle.

Interestingly, products that have been used in facial home treatments for years, like cucumber and papaya, seem to be fairly close to the skin's own pH. Cucumber is a natural cooler that has antiwrinkling benefits, while papaya is rich in natural enzymes and helps slough off dead cells.

You will find, as I have over the years, that many of the most expensive and highly touted skin and hair care products are stripping your acid mantle and leaving you open to bacteria as well as dryness, itchiness, and blotchy complexion. All of these thrive on an alkaline medium. When the skin is acidic, it seems to draw more blood to the surface and can extract nutrients more easily, giving your complexion a healthy glow, which communicates health and vitality. A pale skin may be a sign that your acid mantle needs a little tender loving care.

How can you help to maintain the acid mantle? Combine 1 part apple cider vinegar to 8 parts water. Use it as a toner after washing to keep your facial skin soft, supple, and rosy. You can also rinse your hair with it after shampooing to help keep your scalp free of dandruff. Apple cider vinegar can easily become your most valued cosmetic beautifier. Try pouring one cup full-strength apple cider vinegar into your bath water to relieve sore muscles and overall body dryness and itchiness. Some folk medicine enthusiasts swear that apple cider vinegar taken straight will shrink varicose veins and heal scars.

Beauty Basic Truth #5: Water

Water is an absolute must when it comes to having ageless beauty. Since your body is made up of about 70 percent water, you'll need a constant supply (up to ten or twelve eight-ounce glasses a day) to keep your tissues hydrated, dewy, and youthful. Dehydration shows up as wrinkles and dry, dull, lined skin. It is extremely important to drink filtered water to avoid xenoestrogenic chlorine and to neutralize bacteria found in most municipal water supplies. You can also buy alkaline- and electrolyte-enhanced water that is not only optimum for hydration but is also beneficial in neutralizing the acidic wastes from the detoxification process. (See the Resource section for more information.)

Beauty Basic Drills

Before advancing to tips and routines for your age and stage of life, here are a few basic drills to help you develop a strong, beauty foundation. Look for skin care lines that are organic and as free of petrochemicals as possible.

Drill 1: Cleanse, Tone, and Moisturize

Everybody at every age and stage of life should do the basics twice a day. Always be sure to choose products from natural, nonpetrochemical lines suitable for your skin type.

- Proper cleansing will rid your skin of dirt and impurities—especially important with the amount of environmental pollutants you're encountering each day. Apply a cleanser suitable for your skin type, and use it in the morning (to eliminate wastes on your skin's surface created during the night) and at bedtime (to remove bacteria, oils, and dirt accumulated throughout the day).

- Toning each day helps your skin feel fresh and moist. Toners eliminate any debris left on your skin after cleansing or using a mask or even from your tap water. You might want to leave it in the refrigerator so when you splash it on your face, you'll feel revitalized. Make sure your toner or astringent is alcohol free, or it could irritate and dry your skin.

- Moisturizing your skin—regardless of your skin type—guards your skin from bacteria, makeup, smog, and so forth. Daily moisturizers also fatten up the cells of your skin, lock in moisture, and help your skin feel smooth and silky.

Drill 2: Exfoliate and Apply Masks

For glowing skin, add this drill to your routine about once or twice a week.

- Exfoliation sloughs off those nasty dead skin cells that can lead to blackheads, blemishes, dryness, and wrinkles. Scrubbing also stimulates your circulation to give you a radiant, healthy-looking glow. You can use or make scrubs from a number of items like almond meal, cornmeal, hazelnut meal, jojoba beads or meal, and other grains known to slough off dead skin cells. Make a point to choose gentle exfoliants. (If you have sensitive skin or have broken capillaries, skip this part.)

- Facial masks tighten pores, restore moisture, balance oil, and nurture your skin. Apply the mask and take advantage of the typical ten- to fifteen-minute wait by lying down or listening to some soothing music. Make sure to follow this treatment with a toner and moisturizer.

Drill 3: Use Topical Essential Oils

Essential oils give you a beautifying double whammy. They're good for your skin and hair, plus they're good for your soul.

- With every breath you take, aromas, scents, and smells travel up your nostrils and to your lungs. They send a sensory communiqué through one of two olfactory nerves to the limbic system in your brain. At that point the limbic system, which affects feelings and memories, relays the message to the rest of your body, stimulating your response to the memo. You might want to use a vaporizer to enliven a room's fragrance. For relaxation, try lavender or sandalwood. If you want a more refreshing essence, use citrus scents such as lemon and orange.

- Find the best-quality, pure essential oils, not synthetics. These higher-quality oils are either extracted from herbs, fruits, and flowers via a steam distillation process or, in the case of citrus fruits, are pressed. Shop at your local health food store or herb store so you can be sure the essential oils you are purchasing do not contain water or alcohol and haven't undergone a chemical or toxic process involving carbon dioxide or solvents. Because the oils are so concentrated (more than fifty times more potent that the original plant from which they were derived), just one drop is usually sufficient. So please don't get into that thinking that if a little is good a lot is better. (See the Resources section for mail order suppliers of quality essential oils, under Aromatherapy.)

- Always dilute an essential oil in a cream or carrier oil. My favorite carrier oil is jojoba because it's naturally moisturizing and stable. I strongly recommend that you do not choose oils made from mineral oil (such as baby oil). These oils are petroleum byproducts and are known to clog your pores as well as have a reduced absorption rate.

- Store essential oils in glass. They'll damage plastic, and you'll have more xenoestrogens to deal with.

Once you've got the basics, you're ready for the next step. I've given you a variety of quick fixes that combine cutting-edge science with healing wisdom passed down through the ages, ranging from mineral and herbal supplement aids for various conditions to my favorite home cosmetic remedies. Remember to read tips and routines listed under ages and stages other than your own, because many of today's beauty problems cross age lines. Also, please note that some of the suggested nutrients may already be included in the basic programs outlined for your specific age and stage.

Natural Tips and Beauty Routines for Every Age

Teens and Twenties

Acne Vulgaris

- Say good-bye to sugar. Refined sugar acts more like a drug that our bodies need to detoxify than like a nutrient-supplying food. In fact, sugar has no nutrients. Important skin nutrients such as chromium, manganese, cobalt, zinc, and magnesium are stripped away in sugar refining, and our bodies actually have to use their own mineral reserves just to digest it.

- Take adrenal-supporting supplements like the B-complex vitamins, vitamin C, and an adrenal gland extract. Acne that is brought on by stress may be a result of tired or exhausted adrenal glands. Your adrenals are walnut-sized glands that sit atop your kidneys and perform many tasks in order to keep you alert and healthy.

- Stay away from margarine and all foods that contain hydrogenated oils. Hydrogenated oils interfere with hormones known as prostaglandins, which keep skin healthy and pimple free.

- Think zinc, the beauty mineral highly regarded in treating acne; it has healing, cell-regenerating, skin-calming properties. Take 25 to 50 mg. in the form of zinc picolinate. And be sure to eat zinc-rich foods such as red meat, seafood, and pumpkin seeds.

- Vitamin B_6 (pyridoxine) is notorious for stopping pimples in their tracks. Known as the antidermatitis factor, vitamin B_6 taken in dosages of 50–200 mg. per day will help metabolize fats and fatty acids and balance oil production in the skin.

- Pick up a probiotic (friendly flora that support the GI tract) formula, if you're not taking one already, to restore good bacteria to a sugar-depleted GI tract, especially since sugar feeds yeast and bacteria, which have a negative effect on the skin. Make sure the daily dose

of your probiotic (a combination of acidophilus and bifidobac-
terium) contains 1–10 billion viable organisms.

- Vitamin A, the beautifying vitamin par excellence, is the ticket for
better skin. Using a dosage between 25,000 IU and 50,000 IU per
day for three or four months under the care of a qualified health
practitioner can help fight acne. The water-soluble, or palmitate,
form is probably more absorbable if fat metabolism is problematic,
which can be the case if you're suffering from acne. Don't take
more than 50,000 IU per day unless you're under the care of a
physician. If you're trying to get pregnant or already are pregnant,
keep your vitamin A intake down to 10,000 IU, because the vitamin
can affect fetus development. Beta-carotene may be more ideal if
you're pregnant, since it doesn't interfere with the developing
fetus.

- Limit salty foods and seafood high in iodine. Many people are
iodine sensitive, resulting in the creation of pimples, so it's wise to
limit the intake of these foods.

- Take a supplement of 500–1,000 mg. of L-glutamine up to three
times a day to help with those sugar cravings. L-glutamine converts
to glutamic acid in the brain, which is a house for your energy
source, glucose. This nutrient is also good for hypoglycemic individuals.

- One of my all-time favorite remedies is good old calamine lotion.
It's an outstanding zit zapper. No wonder, since the calamine lotion
is rich in zinc.

- Studies have shown that dabbing a little tea tree oil is as effective
as benzoyl peroxide in treating acne breakouts.

- Try also the following homeopathic remedies: bromium, especially
when there are boils on face and arms; Hepar sulph calcarean
(Hahnemann's calcium sulphide), which targets abscesses; and
Kali bromatum, useful for acne that is accompanied by itching on
the face and chest.

- And finally, there are over-the-counter topical products that contain benzoyl peroxide, sulfur, salicylic acid, or the alpha hydroxies, which have been known to help prevent breakouts and cause red marks to fade.

Oily Skin

- Add a drop of cypress, geranium, or lemon essential oil to your moisturizer for oily skin.

Sensitive Skin

- Vitamin C is one of the top nutrients for your skin. You can take it as a supplement (500–3,000 mg. per day), or use it topically. It can also help retard wrinkles and premature aging.

- The bioflavonoids—substances that have powerful antioxidant ability—are marvelous skin builders. Consider taking Pycnogenol®, a substance with 85 percent bioflavonoid concentration that improves skin and blood vessel health. The usual dosage is 1 mg. per pound of body weight, and it works wonders. Grape seed extract is another source of antioxidant nutrients for sensitive skin that specifically inhibit collagen- and elastin-attacking enzymes, resulting in stronger collagen production.

- Many of my clients swear by their weekly masks of milk of magnesia. It disinfects, soothes, and absorbs excess oil and reduces irritation.

- Exfoliate dead skin cells with alpha hydroxy and beta hydroxy acids. (Caution: exfoliation may exaggerate sun sensitivity. Be sure to use a sunscreen outdoors.) Try gently exfoliating your skin with a mixture of good old-fashioned Cetaphil Skin Cleanser and baking soda. Mix 1–2 teaspoons of baking soda with 1–2 tablespoons of a gentle cleanser like Cetaphil.

- Hydrate skin with water-based, oil-free lotions that contain ingredients (for example, humectants) that help bind moisture to the skin and keep it supple, such as hyaluronic acid, ceramides, and lactic acid.

- Try an aromatherapy facial oil recipe for sensitive skin that really works: Take a clean container and add 1 ounce of jojoba oil, 3 drops neroli oil, 2 drops rose oil, and 2 drops sandalwood oil. Gently turn the container upside down several times or roll it between your hands for a few minutes to blend. Apply several drops to your face twice daily, after cleansing and toning.

- Add a couple drops of jasmine, rosewood, or sandalwood essential oil to your moisturizer to ease sensitive skin.

Facial Hair

- A lack of natural progesterone can create excess facial hair, no matter what your age or stage of life. In the teens and twenties, a lack of ovulation in a skipped period can cause the adrenal cortex to secrete the androgen (steroid) hormone androstenedione as an alternative chemical precursor for the manufacture of progesterone. This steroid is associated with some male characteristics, one of which is male-pattern baldness. But when your progesterone level is raised with natural progesterone cream, your androstenedione level will gradually decline and the excess facial hair will become finer and begin to disappear. For women in their teens and twenties, ¼ teaspoon natural progesterone cream (20 mg.) should be applied once or twice daily beginning on the twelfth day after the first day of the menstrual flow through the twenty-sixth day, stopping during the period.

- In older women (fifty and above) who are no longer menstruating, estrogen dominance can create a progesterone deficiency, resulting in excessive hair growth and facial whiskers. For women in this age group, ¼ teaspoon natural progesterone cream should be applied once or twice daily for a maximum of twenty-five consecutive days, resuming after a five-day break. (See the Resources section for suggestions on progesterone cream.)

- Too much sugar or carbohydrate intake (white flour bagels, muffins, pasta, and bread) can produce excessive facial hair. Carbohydrates increase the secretion of insulin, a hormone that can trigger the adrenals to secrete the androgens testosterone and androstenedione, which are responsible for hair growth on the face.

- Burdock root, a time-honored blood cleanser, also detoxifies the liver, ultimately aiding in the balancing of the high levels of testosterone and androstenedione associated with excessive hair growth. Take one capsule or thirty drops of tincture with each meal for up to two months.

Split Ends

- Zinc to the rescue! This super supplement discourages the conditions that create split ends in your hair. Include at least 20 to 50 mg. per day.

- Panthenol is a component of vitamin B_5 found in nutritional yeast and wheat germ. It helps cells to proliferate and protects and thickens hair. Panthenol acts as a healing agent in skin care, helps to prevent split ends, and smooths the cuticles of hair. It actually increases the hair's diameter for fuller, thicker hair, and is added to many hair-care products currently on the market.

Beautiful Bones

- The teens and twenties are the most crucial years to focus on developing good bones for later in life. According to research by Guy Abraham, M.D., magnesium is most critical for strong, healthy bones. It should be balanced with calcium in about a 2:1 ratio in favor of magnesium (I recommend 500 mg. of calcium from food or supplements with 800–1,000 mg. of magnesium). And you'll also need to get proper amounts of other calcium-building nutrients, such as vitamin D, zinc, manganese, boron, and vitamin C.

- Most important at this age, stay away from the calcium zappers: sugar, coffee, soft drinks, and alcohol. These culprits severely impede your body's ability to properly absorb and use bone-building nutrients. Plus the carbonation in soft drinks neutralizes hydrochloric acid, which impedes the absorption of calcium, protein, and magnesium.

- Although this is contradictory to the estrogen-dominant theme I have discussed earlier, some research suggests that America's exercise craze is leaving some women with very low estrogen reserves, which is further compounded by the xenoestrogens that occupy the natural estrogen receptor sites. As Mom always said, "Everything in moderation," and that includes exercise. Lack of body fat (especially prevalent with ballet dancers and athletes) can cause your body to stop producing natural estrogen and using calcium, which is dependent upon estrogen, creating the possibility of osteoporosis in the teens and twenties.

Thirties and Forties

Lines under the Eyes

- To smooth fine lines, here's an old-time favorite: Brew a strong tea of line-softening eye bright herb (available in health stores). Dunk gauze into tea. Apply moistened gauze over eyelids for thirty minutes. (You'll need to dunk the gauze periodically into the tea to keep it moist.) It's best to lie down while doing this treatment.

- Here's another great tip for erasing facial lines. Mix one egg white with enough heavy cream so the preparation spreads easily. Apply to clean skin. Let the liquid dry on the skin for about thirty minutes, and wash off with warm water. Amazing!

- Patting a vitamin E–containing cream gently into the lines has been known to do wonders. You may also break open a capsule of 400 IU of vitamin E and get the same benefits.

- Some swear that a dab of castor oil on the lines under your eyes can work wonders.

- A prescription vitamin-A derivative called Renova has been shown to reduce lines under the eyes as well as wrinkles on the face. Alpha hydroxy acid lotions work in a similar way. Look for products with a 5 percent to 8 percent concentration of alpha hydroxies, having a pH level of 3 to 4. If lines still persist, consider a glycolic peel or erbium laser resurfacer, which can stimulate collagen growth and tighten skin.

Puffy Eyes

- Steep herbal tea bags in hot water for twenty minutes and then refrigerate. Place the cold, wet tea bags under your eyes. The tea bags contain inflammation-reducing tannic acid, which quickly combats puffiness. Chamomile tea is particularly refreshing and toning for the skin tissues around the eye.

- Cucumber masks soothe eyes. Place thin slices of cucumber on eyes. Cover with a hot washcloth for twenty minutes.

- Make some rose hips tea (strong would be better), and plunk two cotton pads in the tea. Let them stand for a few minutes, then relax and put the pads on your eyelids. Not only will the tea help reduce the puffiness, it will also feel refreshing and help tighten your skin.

Dark Circles

- Place half a fresh fig over each eye to help erase dark circles. Leave on for twenty minutes.

- Dark circles are often a signal of parasites or allergies. I suggest removing all common allergens from your diet, including wheat products, dairy, and chocolate. It may also be extremely helpful to go on a parasite cleanse (see Resources for products). In over a decade of experience, I've never seen a person with persistent dark circles who didn't also have an intestinal parasite infestation.

Wrinkles

- Magnesium is one of the most important hydrating and calming nutrients for beautiful skin (400–800 mg. per day). It works in conjunction with vitamin B_6 and antioxidant nutrients like Pycnogenol® or grapefruit seed extract in preventing wrinkles.

- Having a vitamin A deficiency can lower the mucopolsaccharides in your skin and consequently speed up aging. A maximum dose of 25,000 IU of vitamin A daily helps fight wrinkles and maintain internal moisture. And be sure to eat foods rich in vitamin A, like carrots, sweet potatoes, leafy green vegetables, peaches, and apricots. (If you're trying to get pregnant or already are pregnant, keep your vitamin A intake down to 10,000 IU, because the vitamin can affect fetus development. Beta-carotene may be more ideal if you're pregnant, since it doesn't interfere with the developing fetus.)

- Pierce a capsule of 200 IU natural vitamin E oil (d-alpha toco-pherol or mixed tocopherols), and rub it gently on the wrinkled area consistently every night before going to bed. Also wonderful on cuticles.

- Try a yogurt toning mask to tighten and tone your skin. Combine ½ cup plain yogurt with a little fresh lemon juice. Apply for twenty minutes until dry.

- For softening wrinkles, target spots with Retina A or Renova, or Retinol (a vitamin A derivative), which may be less irritating for those with more sensitive skin, and is found in some cosmetic creams. Many individuals find Retina A or Renova irritating so be careful. Try it every other day for a couple of weeks.

Collagen Loss

- Take 500 to 3,000 mg. of vitamin C daily to help your skin build and maintain collagen. And you could pick up one of the vitamin C topicals as well to fight free radicals.

- The amino acid proline also rebuilds collagen.

Dry Skin

- A vitamin A deficiency can cause dry skin as well as reduce the mucopolsaccharides in the skin, which accelerates the skin's aging process. To add luster to the skin, hair, and nails, take 25,000 IU of vitamin A daily. (If you're trying to get pregnant or already are preg-nant, keep your vitamin A intake down to 10,000 IU, since it can affect fetus development. Beta-carotene may be more ideal if you're pregnant, since it doesn't interfere with the developing fetus.)

- Use vitamin C serum in the morning (see Resources for products). It'll protect you from sun and environmental damage by neutraliz-ing those free radicals that lead to premature aging, sunspots, and discoloration.

- Give skin a healthy glow. Try this old-fashioned recipe straight from my grandmother, who always had flawless skin. Her secret was very simple: two parts rosewater to one part glycerin. After cleansing skin, apply a few drops all over face as a toner and to rejuvenate.

- How about giving yourself a mayonnaise facial? Go to the health food store and pick up some mayonnaise and massage it into the skin for fifteen minutes. Rinse thoroughly in tepid water.

- Make a mask of dry-grind oatmeal and add a whipped whole egg. Massage into face and let stand for five or ten minutes. Rinse with warm, then cool, water. The oatmeal acts as an abrasive and the egg as a protein.

- Here's a great mask to try: Beat together 1 egg, 1 tablespoon milk, and 1 teaspoon honey. Apply to face and neck to harden. May stay on as long as you like. Remove with warm water, followed by cold.

- This one dates back to Cleopatra. Beat together 1 egg white, 1 teaspoon spirits of camphor, 1 heaping tablespoon skim milk powder, and a few drops of mint flavoring. Apply a thin film of odorless castor oil to your skin. Follow with a thick layer of mask. Lie flat for fifteen minutes. Wash off with warm water, followed by witch hazel. By the way, witch hazel helps to restore correct pH balance.

- Be sure to use lotions having sunscreen protection.

- Try an aromatherapy facial mask for dry or mature skin: In the palm of your hand, blend 2 drops of sandalwood oil and 1 drop frankincense oil with 2 teaspoons of honey. Apply the mask to clean skin. Relax for fifteen minutes, then rinse thoroughly. Use this mask once a week.

- Add a couple of drops of essential oils such as neroli, lavender, or jasmine to your moisturizer to soften dry skin.

Freckles and Brown Spots

- Brownish spots are often the result of overexposure to the sun. So remember to use sunscreens to stop any future spots from occurring.

- The antioxidant vitamins C and E, and selenium, as well as glutathione and grape seed extract, help to prevent freckles and brown spots.

- Brown spots appearing on hands, face, arms, and other parts of the body that are not attributed to excess sun may be a sign of adrenal insufficiency. In addition to reducing stress and taking natural progesterone, try rubbing 400 IU of vitamin E or castor oil on spots, once in the morning and once in the evening.

- Cucumber masks help bleach freckles and lighten brown spots. Place thin slices of cucumber on face. Cover with a hot wash-cloth for twenty minutes. Remove slices and rinse with cold water.

- Try lemon juice, an old-time remedy for bleaching. Lemon skins rubbed over the hands will help bleach or lighten spots. Buttermilk with its natural lactic acid may also help.

Petachiae (Elevated Red Spots)

- Cleanse your liver. Liver toxicity can be the underlying culprit to your having those red pinpoints that appear then disappear on your body. Be sure to care for your liver every spring using the detox methods discussed in chapters 3 and 4 to ensure that it's function-ing normally and not becoming overloaded by toxins, which can eventually erupt on your skin.

- Maintain a healthy liver by taking a daily high-fiber supplement containing a synergistic balance of fiber, digestive enzymes, and intestinal flora to keep your colon and liver operating properly. Choose one that also provides liver-supporting and cleansing herbs like Irish moss, buckthorn, butternut, and peppermint, or milk thistle, artichoke, and burdock root. (Please see Resources section.)

Pale Skin

- If you happen to be as pale as a plate of tofu, you might be anemic. Iron prevents anemia, which causes a pale, drawn complexion. Red meat (the darker the color, the greater the iron content) is what I suggest adding to your diet. Other iron-rich foods are organic liver, beans, eggs, spinach, and broccoli.

- Pale or sallow skin usually reveals a lack of acidity in the body—a sign that the acid mantle has been disturbed. Use a vinegar wash, which will soon bring color back to the skin.

- Try the following simple mask, which has been known to help with circulation: Apply buttermilk or milk of magnesia as a mask. Wash off after twenty minutes.

Enlarged Facial Pores

- Control that excessive oil and tighten facial pores with a topical vitamin B complex, which is water soluble. You may want to put some liquid protein (try your hairdresser or health food store) on the area to help strengthen the muscles around the pore itself, often a cause of large pores. Protein also helps tighten the pores.

- Witch hazel, which acts as a facial tightener, can be smoothed on during the daytime. For faster results try rubbing your face with an ice cube wrapped in a cloth.

- Try a facial mask made with one beaten egg white mixed with lemon juice to tighten pores.

- Here's an innovative mask that really works: Mix almond meal with enough water to make a paste. Apply to pores for twenty minutes. Rinse and apply witch hazel.

Blotchy Skin

- Skin blotches may be a sign of hormone imbalance, so you'll want to balance the copper and estrogen overload by increasing progesterone and zinc and taking a copper-free multivitamin. For women in their thirties and forties, I recommend using a topical progesterone cream in the amount of ¼ teaspoon (20 mg.) once or twice a day beginning on the seventh day after the first day of menstrual flow through the twenty-seventh day and stopping during the period. In addition to taking a copper-free multiple supplement, up your intake of zinc-rich foods, such as organic eggs, organic beef, and pumpkin seeds.

- One woman who suffered from blotchy skin for many years suddenly found a solution to her problem. After cleansing her skin, she splashed 1 part cider vinegar to 8 parts distilled water on her face twice a day and allowed it to dry. It worked because the increased acidity in her skin drew more blood to her face, evening out her skin tone.

• Try applying a compress of cold whole milk to irritated areas before using a moisturizer.

Facial Hair

• For women in their thirties and forties, a lack of ovulation in a skipped period can cause the adrenal cortex to secrete the androgen (steroid) hormone androstenedione as an alternative. This steroid is associated with male characteristics such as male-pattern baldness. When the progesterone level is raised with natural progesterone cream, your androstenedione level will decline and eventually the facial hair will become finer and disappear. I recommend taking a natural progesterone cream in the amount of ¼ teaspoon applied once or twice daily beginning on the seventh day after the first day of menstrual flow through the twenty-seventh day and stopping during the period.

• Too much sugar or carbohydrate intake (white flour, bagels, muffins, pasta, and bread) can produce excessive facial hair. Carbohydrates increase the secretion of insulin, a hormone that can trigger the adrenals to secrete the androgens testosterone and androstenedione, which are responsible for hair growth on the face.

Dull Hair

• Drab-looking hair may need a vitamin A boost and/or foods rich in this essential nutrient, such as brightly colored vegetables and fish-liver oil. Also try adding vitamin E (400–800 IU) to your regimen for color and brightness as well as more choline, a B vitamin that metabolizes fat (up to 1,000 mg. a day). Be sure your daily multiple vitamin contains niacinamide (B_3) to give your hair shine. Also taking the trace mineral silica can help your hair have luster.

• Bump up your protein absorption by taking two HCL (10 grains) and pepsin (2 grains) capsules with every protein meal of meat, fish, poultry, or beans.

- A component of vitamin B_5 (pantothenic acid) called panthenol helps add volume to your hair, making it thicker and fuller. It also helps in preventing split ends. Wash your hair with a shampoo containing panthenol for wonderful sheen.

- MSM—methylsulfonylmethane—is a nutritional supplement containing ⅓ sulfur, nature's beauty mineral for keeping hair, skin, and nails healthy. Take 500 mg. three times daily. MSM is available in local health food stores.

- Here's an easy dandruff scalp treatment for you to try. Get a container and mix 2 ounces jojoba oil with 3 drops tea tree oil, 6 drops rosemary oil, 4 drops cedarwood oil, and 3 drops pine oil. Apply some of the mixture to your scalp and massage gently. Leave it on for thirty minutes or even overnight. You can then shampoo your hair with a dandruff-reducing shampoo. Repeat the treatment several times a week, as needed.

Dry Hair

- Essential oils for dry hair: Add a couple of drops of essential oils of lavender, rosemary, or cedarwood to your shampoo or conditioner.

Oily Hair

- Add a couple of drops of these essential oils to your shampoo or conditioner: cypress, lemon, juniper, or pine for oily hair. If you have dandruff, add a couple of drops of tea tree oil to your shampoo or conditioner.

- Taking 50–200 mg. daily of vitamin B_6 helps balance oil glands.

Hair Loss

- Biotin is most effective in preventing hair from falling out. Find a high-dose biotin product (I suggest 5 mg.).

- Use a natural, topical progesterone cream. Use it every day for twenty-five days, and then stop for five days during menstruation. (Please see Resources section.)

- Since hair is 98 percent protein, make sure you are eating enough lean fish and poultry. But remember, protein can't be digested without sufficient hydrochloric acid (HCL). I recommend taking two HCL (10 grains) and pepsin (2 grains) capsules a day with protein meals of meat, fish, and poultry.

- Here's a folklore remedy that works: Mix ½ cup of cayenne pepper with a pint of 100-proof vodka. Every day for two weeks, shake the mixture several times and then strain. You now have liquid capsicum, and cheaper than it would cost to buy. (Don't drink it.) Each morning and evening, apply the mixture to the thinning scalp areas. Within five or six weeks, be on the lookout for new sprouts.

- Add a couple of drops of essential oils like clary, sage, rosemary, or ylang-ylang to your shampoo or conditioner.

Mouth Corner Cracks and Whistle Lines

- Cracks around the corners of the mouth as well as cracked lips can be signs of B_2 or riboflavin deficiency. Try supplementing with vitamin B_2, not more than 50 mg. a day. (The copper-free multiple I recommend contains a total of 50 mg. of B_2 daily.)

Brittle Nails

- Cut the carbs, and get some protein back into your diet! A diet that is too high in carbohydrates and low in protein can cause thinning skin and brittle nails. Protein fortifies your nails—and remember, your nails are made of 98 percent protein. Good sources of protein in the diet include lean meat, fish, chicken, eggs, and beans. Eggs contain the beautifying amino acid cysteine, which contains sulfur and binds the strains of nail protein (keratin) together to give you strong nails.

- An MSM (methylsulfonylmethane) supplement, which contains one-third sulfur, should also be taken, since it is one of nature's beauty minerals for healthy hair, skin, and nails. Take 500 mg. three times daily. MSM is available in local health food stores.

- Also be sure to take at least two HCL (10 grains) and pepsin (2 grains) capsules a day with protein meals of meat, fish, and poultry.

- The right kind of fat in the diet works wonders for poor nail health. Take 2,000 mg. of GLA capsules per day to help restore nails back to health.

- Take 1–2 tablespoons each day of flaxseed oil or a combination of flaxseed oil and evening primrose oil.

- Despite the popular belief that gelatin is not good for nails because of its limited amino acids, I strongly believe and have seen for myself how it can be extremely helpful for strengthening nails. Gelatin contains mucopolsaccharides and the amino acid proline, which regenerate tissue on a cellular level and support collagen.

- Nails are porous and can absorb lots of water. In fact, your nails can absorb 20 percent to 25 percent of their own weight in water. This is why immersing nails in water takes its toll and causes them to become brittle. Try a waxy lip balm from a health food store to seal and waterproof nails.

- Add a B-complex tablet to your diet, 100 mg. twice a day for at least two months.

- Supplement with 2.5–5 mg. of biotin per day to get nails back to health. In one landmark study alone, veterinarians gave high dosages of biotin to horses, which resulted in a marked difference in the strength of their hooves.

- Apple cider vinegar applied directly to nails has been known to strengthen them.

Nail Fungus

- Soak nails in 3 percent hydrogen peroxide for 1–2 minutes twice daily.

- Applying tea tree oil topically has been known to clear the fungus among us.

- Also try dipping a cotton swab in bleach and dabbing it under your nails.

Dry Nails

- Living in Montana, where fighting dry nails has been the bane of my existence, I've learned to keep a purse-sized container of nail moisturizer with me wherever I go. I apply it to my nails throughout the day. Avoid petroleum jelly, which is a xenohormone. Choose a moisturizer with lanolin, which penetrates deep into the skin and nail tissues, allowing them to rehydrate from within without clogging pores.

- If your splitting nails and cracked fingertips are serious problems, pure lanolin is superb.

- Restore moisture by choosing products such as hypoallergenic lanolin, vitamin E oil, and wheat germ oil. The best time to apply them is at night.

Spider Veins

- Drink a lot of water to keep your skin cool by allowing it to sweat. That'll help prevent the eruption of tiny capillaries in your face when it is overheated and flushed.

- Pycnogenol® is an outstanding source of procyaniddic oligomers (PCOs), a specific type of bioflavonoid that strengthens capillaries and helps to stabilize collagen. Take 1 mg. per pound of body weight daily.

- Many women swear by topical vitamin K, which can diminish the appearance of spider veins and sometimes cause them to fade.

Varicose Veins

- Here's an old English and Scottish folk medicine beauty secret for shrinking varicose veins: Apply apple cider vinegar straight out of the bottle to the varicose veins evening and morning. Shrinking of the veins should be noticed in about one month.

- You may want to try 50 mg. three times daily of a standardized extract known as aescin, from natural horse-chestnut seed, to build up those blood vessel walls. Available in health food stores and some drugstores, oral supplements and topical creams help lower fluid leakage and aches associated with varicose veins.

- Increase the amount of bioflavonoids and vitamin C (in citrus and supplement) available in your diet, since they are each great helpers in strengthening your blood vessel walls.

Fifties, Sixties, and Beyond

Beautiful Bones

- A dietary supplement known as ipriflavone in the amount of 600 mg. or 200 mg. three times daily is a nonhormonal prevention and treatment for osteoporosis. Used in conjunction with magnesium, calcium, vitamin C, vitamin D, vitamin K, boron, and zinc, ipriflavone provides the most effective bone-building support, increasing bone density 3–9 percent.

Thinning Hair

- Biotin is great for helping to stop hair from thinning or falling out.

- Use a natural progesterone cream. Use it once a day for twenty-five days and then take a break for five days to two weeks and resume again. The recommended dosage is ¼ teaspoon (20 mg.).

- Since hair is 98 percent protein, make sure you are eating enough eggs, lean fish, and poultry. However, protein needs hydrochloric acid (HCL) to be properly digested. I suggest taking two HCL (10 grains) and pepsin (2 grains) capsules a day with protein meals. The amino acids L-cysteine and methionine can also help.

- If you're still on that low-fat kick, you may lack sulfur, which in turn can lead to hair loss, especially in women. You might want to try taking a sulfur-rich supplement (up to 5 grams a day) to help put a halt to thinning hair or hair loss. Also include sulfur-rich foods such as eggs and meat in your diet.

- Silicon, along with sulfur, is called the "beauty mineral" because it's essential for the growth of thick luxurious hair and for having a natural sheen. The chief sources of silicon are steel-cut oats, apples, honey, avocados, artichokes, and sunflower seeds.

- Good circulation is needed to feed the hair. So be sure to get all the nutrients that build healthy red blood cells and keep arteries clear: antioxidants, essential fatty acids, vitamins B_6, folic acid, and vitamin B_{12}. And, of course, exercise is also important to keep circulation healthy.

- A deficiency of the B vitamin biotin causes thinning hair as well as hair loss.

Problem Gums

- Japanese research on CoQ10 shows that taking 30–90 mg. daily is extremely helpful with bleeding gums, deterioration of the gums, and loosening teeth.

- To ensure the connective tissues holding your gums together are properly formed, you'll need sufficient amounts of vitamin C. Sometimes taking as much as 5–7 grams a day is helpful.

- Magnesium again to the rescue! A deficiency of magnesium produces swollen and sore gums, which improve when magnesium is added to the diet.

Dry Skin

- Vitamin A deficiency reduces the mucopolsaccharides in the skin, which accelerates the skin's aging process and causes dry skin. Take 25,000 IU of vitamin A daily to give skin, hair, and nails a luster.

- Try a natural moisturizer made of pure hypoallergenic lanolin.

- Here's my favorite recipe for an extra-rich moisturizer. Take an unscented body cream, add 4 capsules of vitamin A (25,000 IU) and 10 capsules of vitamin E (100 IU), and mix them together. I use this concoction daily to give my skin super-antioxidant protection from the outside.

- Be certain to include a vitamin B complex to help regulate your body's metabolic functions. B vitamins are also part of the prosthetic group of enzymes vital for skin cell respiration.

- Overcome dry or rough skin with foods containing fatty acids from the omega-3 and -6 families like salmon, nuts, and seeds. Also known as vitamin F, these fatty acids are wonderful defenders against skin problems such as eczema. Flaxseed oil, borage, and evening primrose oil can be taken in supplement form. Borage can be applied topically.

- For dry hands, try creating your own hand cream. Mix 1 fluid ounce olive oil with a pinch of tartar. Add ½ pint rosewater and a pinch of borax. Mix well and rub into hands.

Tired Eyes

- Here's a favorite as old as the hills that really works. Dissolve 1 teaspoon of boric acid in 1 pint of boiling water and allow to cool. Soak some cotton wool pieces in the liquid and keep in a cool place, such as your fridge. Place the swabs onto your eyes for a few minutes.

Special Conditions

If you're not getting enough beauty rest or are under a lot of stress and have become emotionally distraught, these inward problems can be taking a toll on your looks. So I've also included some tips for these as well as other types of beauty concerns that can arise from time to time.

Insomnia

- Vitamin B_{12} appears to significantly help insomnia. A 3,000-mcg. dose, according to one study, enables people with sleep problems to drift off more easily and to remain asleep for a longer period.

- Try taking 400 mg. of magnesium just before bedtime. It seems to help brain chemistry and promote sleep. (Interestingly, biochemist David Watts taught me that constant waking cycles signal a magnesium deficiency and the inability to go to sleep initially signals a calcium deficiency.)

- If your pineal gland isn't properly releasing melatonin, you will experience disturbances in your sleeping-waking cycles. That's why taking melatonin is often the number one answer. By taking .03 mg. of this physiologically active sleeping pill at bedtime, you may enjoy a restful night's sleep.

- If your system is too acidic, you can't sleep. So try taking ¼ teaspoon sea salt dissolved in 8 ounces of water before bedtime. It will neutralize your system and help promote sleep.

- Exercise during the daytime. Evening exercise increases body temperature and can make it more difficult to fall asleep.

- Get some sunlight. Adjust your internal clock (circadian rhythm) by stepping outdoors for forty-five minutes as soon as you wake up. How about reducing sensory stimulation for an hour or two before bedtime? Cut the TV and the stereo earlier in the evening and you'll sleep better, I've found.

Depression

- Sometimes by controlling blood sugar levels, depression disappears. So you might want to include protein, fat, and some carbohydrates at meals and snack times. Also try removing wheat from your diet. And as recommended in the detox menu programs, continue taking one or two tablespoons of flaxseed oil or a combination of flaxseed oil and evening primrose oil in your daily regimen. It may be helpful in combating depression.

- Consider trying the highly touted St. John's wort, known to help many individuals. Lacking the troublesome side effects of other tricyclic antidepressants, this incredible herb is a serotonin-selective reuptake inhibitor, much like Prozac. Typically, taking 300 mg. three times a day is helpful; be sure to use the standardized extract having 0.3 percent hypericin. You can also take ½ ounce of the dried herb daily as a tea or tincture. (Note: some people may experience a photosensitivity while taking St. John's wort. As with most supplements, it could take up to several weeks before benefits are realized. If you don't feel this herb is working for you, try chasteberry.)

- Also try taking 500 mg. of tyrosine three times every day, which is a precursor to thyroid hormones. Many depressed individuals find they have a hypothyroid condition, so you may want to consider having your thyroid function checked.

- Natural progesterone cream has been known to assist proper thyroid functions. So if you're not using one, consider adding it to your regimen.

- A combination of royal jelly, bee pollen, and bee propolis found in a supplement called Bee's Secret from Purity Products has been found to decrease depression and increase euphoria.

Rashes, Rosacea, and Dermatitis
- I've seen many women obtain outstanding results after using topical or internal progesterone supplements. One of my clients (with a doctor's prescription) took micronized oral progesterone, 100–200 mg. per day, and her rosacea disappeared in just two weeks.

- Rashes, rosacea, and dermatitis may also be related to a hydrochloric acid deficiency (see chapter 5).

Pregnancy Mask
- Dark areas of pigmentation or skin blotches on the face often are signs of copper overload. This unusual pigmentation is most likely to occur during pregnancy, when estrogen and copper levels rise. During this time, some women develop what doctors call a "pregnancy mask," dark areas on the face, especially above the lip and on the lower forehead. As indicated throughout this book, hormone balance can be brought into check by reducing your copper intake (a symptom of estrogen dominance) and cultivating a zinc-rich diet. If you're not eating enough protein, increasing your intake will assist your body in ferreting out the extra copper.

Eczema
- Try colloidal oatmeal products. They provide excellent relief from the burning, soreness, and itching of eczema.

- There's one exceptional product you really should try: a pure hypoallergenic lanolin derived from shorn wool, which penetrates deep into the skin, allowing it to rehydrate from the inside, without clogging pores. It's also good for dry, cracked lips, heels, and elbows as well as dry nails. It's even good for nipples dried out from breast feeding. (See Resources.)

- GLA dosages from 300–500 mg. have been found in clinical studies to clear up eczema.

- Chronic low intake of vitamin A will produce some of the symptoms of eczema, including dry, scaly, and rough skin. The skin typically clears up on a strong supplement program, using a dosage between 25,000 IU and 50,000 IU per day for three or four months under the care of your qualified health practitioner. Remember, higher dosages may become toxic, so don't increase your intake without consulting your physician first. (If you're trying to get pregnant or already are pregnant, keep your vitamin A intake down to 10,000 IU because the vitamin can affect fetus development. Beta-carotene may be more ideal if you're pregnant since it doesn't interfere with the developing fetus.)

- Eczemalike symptoms also develop during a deficiencies of vitamin B_3, vitamin B_{12}, folic acid, biotin, and pantothenic acid.

Psoriasis

- Topical borage oil (puncture a capsule and apply) has been found to heal psoriasis conditions very effectively.

- Zinc deficiencies have been associated with psoriasis. Make sure you are supplementing your diet with at least 25–50 mg. of zinc daily.

- In the Atkins Clinic in New York, psoriasis is treated with large doses of folic acid, ranging from 20 to 40 mg. daily. Although this has not been documented with clinical studies, the Atkins Center has had remarkable results.

- Essential fatty acids are beneficial. Take 1 or 2 tablespoons of flaxseed oil or a combination of flaxseed and primrose oils.

- Olive leaf extract, in a standardized 12 percent extract, can be phenomenal for clearing up psoriasis. The recommended dosage is six capsules a day of 250 mg. olive leaf and 250 mg. standardized extract.

Scars

- By taking the nutritional supplement MSM (methylsulfonylmethane) before surgery, some individuals have noticed reduced scarring. Whether the supplement or topical form is used, it seems not only to reduce scarring, but also to alleviate the accompanying pain. After surgery, it might help subdue scars if you take 2 to 8 grams of MSM daily. (The amount will vary upon your gastrointestinal tolerance.) MSM is available in crystal form from local health food stores.

- Would you believe an onion extract can help erase scars? We already knew that compounds in onions can help lighten up age spots. But the actual extract, allium cepa, has been put in a gel formulation that you can apply to scars. (See Resources.) Apply it twice a day for five to ten minutes. It is supposed to reduce the appearance of scars in just eight weeks.

- Relatively new on the market is an FDA-approved treatment that is said to cause scars (even those you've had for years) to disappear. Previously physicians and even some plastic surgeons used the treatment (a rubberlike material that's actually a silicone sheet) to treat scars on burn victims. It can be found under two brand names (see Resources); you may find them in your local drugstore.

- A tried-and-true remedy for scarring has always been a topical application of vitamin E, 400–800 mg., placed directly on the scar.

- You might try to supplement with an amino acid combination that contains proline—known to support and stabilize collagen production. You can also supplement with proline alone in a 500 mg. capsule; use one twice a day between meals.

Stretch Marks (Striae)

- Our grandmothers used cocoa butter (available in drug and some health stores). They rubbed it on their tummies during pregnancy to reduce stretch marks.

- Remember that skin is mostly protein. If you're deficient in protein or in hydrochloric acid (HCL), which aids your body in assimilating protein, take two HCL (10 grains) and pepsin (2 grains) capsules with every protein meal of meat, fish, poultry, or beans.

Aching Muscles

- A remedy that has been used for decades is taking a hot steaming bath in 1–2 cups of Epsom salts. Rich in magnesium, Epsom salts help to soothe aching muscles.

Sagging Muscles

- Adding more potassium-draining foods to your diet may do the trick, particularly if you're on diuretics or drink tea, coffee, or alcohol. Select foods like parsley, sunflower seeds, almonds, halibut, cod, turkey, mushrooms, chard, spinach, cantaloupe, and avocado. Are you tired or do you feel weak in your muscles? To boost energy levels or endurance, try combining 250–500 mg. potassium aspartate with the same amount of magnesium aspartate.

Cosmetic Surgery

- If you're going in for a face-lift, chemical peel, laser resurfacing, eyelid surgery, or liposuction, adopting a special nutrient-rich routine designed to curtail bruising is strongly recommended. Start the program a week before surgery and continue it for two to three weeks afterward. Your routine should include:

  1. Taking 4 pellets of the homeopathic remedy Arnica (6X) four times a day

  2. Taking 1,000 mg. of bromelain per day

  3. Taking 50 mg. of zinc each day

  4. Taking 500–5,000 mg. of vitamin C daily

  5. Taking 2 mg. of Pycnogenol® per each pound of body weight for one week, then 1 mg. per each pound of body weight thereafter

- If you're undergoing either deep chemical peels or laser resurfacing, be aware that the herpes virus can be stimulated. Take either antiviral medication before or after the procedure, or supplement with 500 mg. of the herpes-fighting lysine.

Breast Augmentation

- If you're interested in "safe" breast enlargement without scars, adhesions, or physical discomfort, there are now all-natural enhancement supplements available made from phytoestrogenic herbs and grains. Many women experience a one- to two-cup size increase within two to seven months. (See Resources.)

You really have come a long way, baby! From deciphering what your body's been telling you to understanding the importance of detoxification and hormonal balance, you've accomplished a great deal in your journey to attaining a living beauty. And now that you're armed with these valuable tips and routines, you can enhance your overall beauty and vitality every day of the year—for the rest of your life. Let's transition by exploring the inner you in the next chapter. Hopefully you will discover the right self-health practice to fully express your own authentic beauty from within. We will be taking the detox experience to a deeper, more meaningful level—just a page away.

9

Detoxing the Inner

I have an everyday religion that works for me:
Love yourself first and everything else falls into line.
LUCILLE BALL

As you clear out physical toxins from your body, it's not uncommon for emotional toxins to surface. Suppressed emotions like anger, fear, grief, and anxiety begin to manifest, and so you may find yourself wanting to continue your detoxification process on deeper levels. Once the physical wastes are gone from your body and harmony is established, from elimination and digestion to hormonal and biochemical balance, you'll have more clarity of thought to communicate feelings that were never expressed or to experience closure of a particular event or relationship.

The whole deep-cleansing process reminds me a little of an onion. After peeling away the delicate outer layers of the detox process, you're ready to cleanse the denser layers, which represent your spiritual, emotional, and mental being. This purging on all levels is not only a common, natural transition in the detoxification process but also an extremely necessary part in your quest for beauty and vitality.

The truth is that many of the problems in your life may be related to unresolved, suppressed feelings about events you experienced. Much like icebergs hidden deep beneath the ocean's surface, these emotions lie submerged in your subconscious, where they stay undetected for years. Fueled by negative energy, they secretly hinder your journey to health, healing, and radiant beauty and swallow up any chance you may have for developing and enjoying good relationships. No matter how hard you try, you can't merely push away or sidestep these emotional icebergs. Unresolved feelings like guilt or anger constantly stir deep inside you and cause you to be overly critical of others and yourself or make you feel upset, irritated, and frustrated most of the time. And all too often your loved ones end up paying the price, becoming the brunt of your unexplained outbursts.

Dissolving these suppressed emotions is the only way to defuse them so you can be free and filled with vitality and a deeper, more appreciative sense of well-being. As a matter of fact, the importance of resolving these emotions has become so widely known that many national newspapers—not just medical journals—are reporting the latest findings on the subject. Take a look at the following facts from an article published in *USA Today* ("Suppressing Emotions May Shorten Your Life," August 10, 1991) that reflect research showing a definite connection between emotions and health.

- Out of forty-eight sixth-grade boys, half suppressed their emotions, while the others freely expressed theirs; one-third of the emotionally suppressed group had asthma, but no one in the emotionally expressive group did.

- A study of 179 men showed that those who had suppressed hostility also had "predicted higher LDL (bad cholesterol)."

- Participants in a forty-one-year study at Johns Hopkins University who didn't express tension and emotion at age twenty were twice as likely to die by age fifty-five than those who freely expressed anxieties.

Showing the link between blood pressure and emotional expression, Dr. Samuel Mann of New York Hospital–Cornell Medical Center reported that patients with hypertension have buried past traumas deeply in their sub-conscious. He believes that often the answer to their stress is not in the here and now but rather in the past they have repressed (*USA Today*, "Hiding Emotions, Hypertension Linked," March 19, 1996). Dr. Johan Denollet of the University of Antwerp, Belgium, agrees with this emotional link theory, suggesting that stress encourages arrhythmia and the narrow-ing of the arteries. He encourages Type D patients (those who typically withhold emotions) to get behavior therapy. Dr. Denollet also found that out of the 303 heart patients he observed over a period of six to ten years, those burying negative emotions had a four-times-higher risk of dying from a heart attack. And in a study of 260 women conducted by researcher Darla Vale of Rush–Presbyterian–St. Luke's Medical Center in Chicago, those having heart problems were more apt to suppress their anger (*USA Today*, "Heart Risk Increases for Stoic Types," March 11, 1996).

You've already learned how your skin talks to you about physical imbalances going on inside your body. Well, the body as a whole has been trying to communicate a bigger picture of what's been going on deep inside that may be at the root of your overall health concerns. All that suppressed anger, hurt, guilt, and resentment are bottled up and immobilizing your immune system. Once you begin to hear and under-stand the inner wisdom of your body, it's time to take some positive steps toward correcting the problem.

A Path to Healing and Inner Beauty

For years I've practiced self-help techniques that have allowed me to achieve a certain degree of success. Meditation has helped to keep me focused and maintain a sense of peace in my life, while speaking affir-mations has helped me to positively program my mind. Since I'm easily motivated by words or intellect, both of these techniques have worked well for me.

But I also know that much of what affects us lies deep within our subconscious, controlling our lives until we learn to release it. I had reached a point in my life where I felt that I had to go beyond my conscious mind and my overactive intellect and detox and renew my inner self, which led me to a seven-day intensive workshop (see Resources for more information on this workshop).

The workshop dealt with core belief systems, healing relationships, one's emotional autobiography, emotional clearing, and a special kind of connected breathing called BodhiSoul breathwork. Although I gained insight from each of the course's focus areas, the breathwork, in which the inhalation is connected smoothly with the exhalation, brought me to a whole new level of awareness. Rather than programming and doing, I learned how to just be. Instead of forcing the river with affirmations, this breathing technique freed me, allowing me to discover and deal with things that had been suppressed, not expressed, in my life. I dealt with experiences that I had no idea were affecting me, like the following episode.

I remember getting on a school bus when I was about eight years old and someone saying to me, "I wish you would smile more, because when you don't you always look like you're going to cry." I had heard that observation from more than one person, and since I was an overly sensitive child, it bothered me so much that I felt like crying. It wasn't until I started practicing connected breathing that I uncovered what lay behind it: unexpressed grief.

The answer finally came to me in a dream that I had recorded in my journal about two weeks before the workshop. I dreamed that I was in an ocean with a long ropelike lifeline, trying to save a male baby by bringing him to shore. In my journal I wrote how somehow this dream was related to my unconscious because I knew that water symbolizes the unconscious. But beyond that realization, I had no idea what the dream was supposed to be telling me until my first connected breathing session.

Toward the end of the breathing session, I began to cry uncontrollably, and suddenly out of nowhere I realized that I was grieving for my long-forgotten baby brother, Stephen Paul, a "blue baby" who died of heart failure when I was four. My dream, two weeks prior, was my unconscious trying to make me recognize and acknowledge the grief I had stuffed away for over forty years. My trying to pull the baby to shore was a way to recognize and acknowledge Stephen Paul's short life. Since I had always tried to be such a good little girl, I had never acknowledged my true sadness for the tragedy, or maybe I was just too young to fully comprehend his death. Interestingly, after the breakthrough, a huge pimple broke out on my cheek area, which in Chinese medicine relates to the lungs, which in turn is related to the emotion of grief. The blemish was a physical sign to me that I had tapped into and released something deep inside.

Flower Remedies

Another practice that has played a major role in coping with stress and other issues in my life as well as in the lives of those around me is the use of flower remedies. The Bach Flower Remedies, developed in the 1930s by Dr. Edward Bach, a British bacteriologist, are extremely helpful for getting through some rather emotionally difficult situations. Bach discovered that flower and herbal remedies transmute the mental and emotional disharmonies linked to physical ills, and he developed a group of thirty-eight such remedies. Perhaps the most revered is Rescue Remedy, a kind of emotional first aid in a bottle. Used in emergency rooms all over the world, Rescue Remedy contains star of Bethlehem (for numbness and trauma), rock rose (for deep panic and terror), impatiens (for tensions and irritability), cherry plum (for fear of going out of your mind), and clematis (for passing out or being out of your body before unconsciousness). Rescue Remedy has gotten my clients and me through many stressful situations, including car accidents, surgeries, divorce proceedings, courtroom appearances, and just plain everyday anxiety and tension. I will never forget how Rescue Remedy, when added to drinking water throughout the day, was my first aid solution several years ago when my dear cousin Gail, whom I was very close to, unexpectedly passed away at the age of forty-two.

A new generation of flower essences has been developed that is helpful in detoxifying the inner. These remedies help to change fundamental patterns of behavior, feel relaxed and renewed, become more balanced during mental or physical stress, enjoy better concentration or mental focus, maximize energy levels, and restore or regenerate energy levels due to emotional or psychological imbalances.

The following formulas are from Botanical Alchemy and may be used together. The formulator, Clifton Harrison, recommends placing three to four drops under the tongue or in a half-filled glass of water. Sip slowly. If you want to remove traces of alcohol used in the extraction process, place the drops in warm water (not hot) and let sit for a few minutes. It's best to use just one formula at a time about four times daily. For chronic or more severe conditions, however, the formula can be taken every five minutes. Keep them away from strong electromagnetic fields such as television sets.

Botanical Alchemy Emotional Remedies

Formula	Description
Athlete's Spirit (Ginseng)	Increases mental focus and precision while adding strength and fluidity to muscles. Contains ginseng, lotus, cayenne, elm, blue flag.
Bright Mornings (Blue Flag)	For creating an upbeat, positive attitude. Good for the blues. Contains blue flag, digitalis, mustard, grindelia.
Calmchild (Chamomile)	Good for calming children after upsets, anger, or disappointment. Transforms negative energy into a renewed sense of innocence and wonder. Contains chamomile, bleeding heart, grindelia, sunflower.
Cleansing Fire (Geranium)	Addresses any hidden emotional or spiritual issue that may lie behind long-standing symptoms. Cleanses mental, physical, and spiritual bodies to release full vitality. Contains geranium, sagebrush, sage, walnut.
Clear Communication (Horehound)	Opens the throat chakra to strengthen the voice and aligns thoughts and expressions. Contains horehound, calendula, peppermint, sage.
Clear Spirit (Lotus)	For relaxed and even respiration, leading to a strong spirit. Relieves blockages on all levels, opens the crown chakra, and enhances awareness in dealing with birth and death issues. Contains lotus, mugwort, sagebrush, blue corn.

Formula	Description
Courage (Garlic)	Dispels fears by enhancing your system's ability to confront and overcome them. Grounding and stabilizing essences lend fortitude and perseverance. Contains garlic, dandelion, St. John's wort, cinnamon basil, chrysanthemum.
Dreams Come True (Sunflower)	Supports clarity of purpose, assertiveness, and opportunity. Contains sunflower, blackberry, ivy, dogwood, wild oat.
Emotional Transformation (Amaranth)	Goes to any emotional source of illness. Contains amaranth, calendula, dandelion, pine, sage, yarrow.
Hidden Issues (Fuchsia)	A powerful blend to bring up hidden, unknown, or deeply suppressed emotions as indicated by sudden feelings of anger, repeated self-sabotage, addictive behavior, or sadness out of proportion to the current situation. Contains fuchsia, bleeding heart, crab apple.
Immune Energy (Echinacea)	Bolsters the immune system and guards against emotional, mental, and environmental toxins. Contains echinacea, chaparral, blackberry.
Inspiration (Indian Paintbrush)	Stimulates imagination and creativity, increases capacity for problem solving. Contains Indian paintbrush, blackberry, basil, nasturtium.
Mental Focus (Sagebrush)	Improves attention and concentration, which, in a larger sense, keep you from repeating the same mistakes. Contains sagebrush, chestnut, angophora.
New Patterns (Aloe Vera)	Helps change the patterns underlying addictive behavior and soothe unruly cravings. Contains aloe vera, juniper, walnut, blue flag, grindelia.
Perfect Balance (Tulip)	Helps integration of mind, body, and spirit that is lost over time. Contains orange, red, pin, white, and violet tulips.
Rapid Recovery (Apricot)	Restores energy when suffering burnout or exhaustion. Contains apricot, cayenne, coffee, sunflower, nasturtium, olive.
Sexual Healing (Jasmine)	Melts frozen emotions and releases sensual and loving nature. Contains jasmine, rose, hibiscus, angophora.

Continued

Formula	Description
Tranquillity (Lavender)	Designed to quiet the mind and emotions for deep serenity and sound sleep. Contains lavender, catnip, cedar, basil.
Transform Anger (Willow)	Helps to recognize and release old resentments and keep irritations from turning into aggression. Contains willow, saguaro, cholla, prickly pear, marigold, walnut.
Trauma (Arnica)	Helps minimize damage from old shocks and injuries and speed healing. Contains arnica, cinnamon, basil, Indian pink, sage.
Unstress (Yarrow)	Balances and soothes physical and mental chaos from overload situations. Contains yarrow, blue flag, elm, impatiens.
Woman's Harmony (Bluestar)	Helps maintain productivity and balance under stress. Contains bluestar, hibiscus, calendula, daffodil.

Every day of my life I practice one or more basic techniques to feed the soul. And you can too. Flower essences, connected breathing, meditation, and affirmation can all help you cleanse your inner self from suppressed emotions that have been clogging up your life. Just keep in mind that the answers to the joy you're seeking are within you, not outside of you. Detoxing your inner channels will lead you to your true self and unlock the passageway to your personal journey with your higher being.

We've explored flower essences in some depth; now let's take a deeper look at connected breathing, meditation, and affirmations.

Connected Breathing:
Linking the Body to the Soul

Breathing is the energy force of life, from the moment you were born to the moment you draw your last breath. You can fast from food and water, but you can't go without breathing. Connected breathing is a simple breathing technique designed to clear mental, emotional, and physical blocks and suppressions, especially those from birth and early childhood experiences. This powerful yet easy technique can enhance every aspect of your being, from the quality of your life and relationships to your sense of kinship with the physical world and your interactions with money and possessions.

The goal of the connected breathing technique is to experience the feelings of a stored event as you breathe, drawing the toxic emotion out of the subconscious. As you practice this technique, you'll feel the emotions of past events just as you did when they first happened. However, when these events originally occurred, you might have felt unsafe or afraid to fully express your feelings and held your breath, thereby burying your emotions somewhere in your subconscious. Working to clear your inner self of these destructive emotions by breathing through them will empower you to make positive life changes and conscious decisions instead of being enslaved by them and letting them determine what will or won't happen in your life.

The Benefits of Connected Breathing

You have everything to gain from practicing connected breathing, which effortlessly—without concentration—allows past memories and their emotions to resurface and release. Here are some of the more specific ways it may help you:

- reduce stress and deeply relax you

- enhance your creativity

- improve your health and give you more energy

- achieve mental clarity

- stabilize your emotions

- attain an overall sense of well-being

Tips for Practicing Connected Breathing

1. Center yourself, let go, and get connected to your higher power.

2. Ask for guidance.

3. Open your mouth wide, and inhale deeply from your abdomen. Then let the breath simply fall away; do not blow out or control it in any way, and don't pause before or after inhaling or exhaling.

4. Breathe fast and full at the beginning to draw energy into the body. You may inhale and exhale through either your nose or mouth, but do not inhale one way and exhale the other.

5. Allow yourself the freedom to fully experience whatever comes up for you. (You cannot consciously plan what your subconscious has in store.)

6. Breathe fast and shallow to speed up and release an emotion or experience that is extremely painful or uncomfortable, if you wish.

7. Breathe slowly and fully to really absorb a loving or joyous moment; you may also want to use this breathing rhythm at the end of your session if it is pleasant.

8. Keep your breaths connected and even; don't hold your breath out of fear or anger.

Meditation: Let It Be

Meditation helps you open up to new, creative ideas and inspires you to find answers to problems. As you meditate, your entire body reaches a point of rest and yet feels revitalized. Even your mind becomes more alert as you learn to tune in to your intuition. And as an overachiever, I find that meditating helps slow me down and keep me focused on what really needs attention in my life.

But there are even more reasons to mediate. Researchers have found that meditation may very well be linked to better health. In 1990 Harvard researchers Herbert Benson and A. Dormar Goodale conducted a study showing that meditation and other forms of relaxation can actually help reduce PMS or menopausal symptoms. Benson also discovered that meditation lowers blood pressure, slows heart rates, and lowers metabolic rates (*Obstetrics and Gynecology*, vol. 75, no. 4, April 1990). And Dr. Bernie Siegel, surgeon and author of *Love, Medicine, and Miracles*, says that people can take an active part in their own cures by incorporating "self-induced healing." He cites a number of case histories of terminally ill patients who were able to heal themselves by meditating and adopting a new attitude, which brought a state of peace into their lives.

The Benefits of Meditation

Deciding to meditate on a regular basis will surely enhance every facet of your life, from your personal and family affairs to your dealings with the rest of the world.

- reduction in PMS and menopause symptoms

- better physical health

- rest for your body

- recharging of your heart, lungs, and nervous system

- increased creativity and mental alertness

- sharper memory

- improved self-image

Tips on Practicing Meditation

A number of different methods have been handed down to us from many cultures, and there is no "right" way to mediate. Meditation can evolve to become as individual as you are. The goal is to quiet the mind and achieve a sustained state of relaxation no matter which method of meditation you choose. I like to listen to nature sounds, like birds singing or water falling. You'll find what works best for you.

The most important thing is to commit yourself to meditating on a regular basis. You might want to try meditating first thing each morning to get yourself centered for the day. Some people have a specific place for their meditation session, typically somewhere comfortable. It can be a special room in your home or outdoors. To really make a difference, your meditation period should last fifteen or twenty minutes. This will allow you enough time to become grounded. And don't be upset if you don't "see" or "feel" anything. It's okay. I don't get flashes of enlightenment or hear mystical bells going off. Meditation for me means becoming still and learning not to push so hard throughout the day. It has taught me that time has its own destiny regardless of my own agenda. And since my motto in my life has always been, "Whatever is worth doing is worth overdoing," meditation has been a tool in helping me learn to go with the proverbial flow. Just remember, your goal is simply to do it because somehow the action alone will help you become more relaxed, peaceful, and centered. Keep in mind that these recommended steps are only one suggested way to meditate.

1. Sit with your back straight, feet planted flat on the floor, palms turned upward.

2. Close your eyes and begin to look inside to that mystical place of energy located at midpoint between your eyebrows.

3. Let any thoughts you have pass by you freely.

4. Concentrate on your breathing, becoming keenly aware of when the air touches your nostrils as you inhale and exhale.

5. Become comfortable with just "being" as you become more centered and quiet inside.

6. Choose a word or phrase that holds special meaning for you—such as "God is love" or "harmony, peace, joy"—and repeat it each time you exhale.

7. Continue your meditation session for five or ten minutes at first, then build to fifteen or twenty minutes or longer.

Affirmation: Creating Positive Energy Within You

An affirmation is a positive word or statement that is spoken in the now and targets what you want to be like in the future. When you repeat it, your mind opens up, and in time the affirmation becomes a part of your being and self-image. Affirmations can help you change your inner attitude and truths, but they cannot alter your outer reality. Remember how we approached beauty and health from the inside out? Cleansing your inner self with all of these self-help techniques works the same way. Affirmations offer you an excellent way to reprogram your thinking. By consciously focusing on your new affirmation, you'll eventually drop old patterns and destructive thoughts.

Divine Guidance author Doreen Virtue, Ph.D., explains in her book that fostering negative attitudes will cause them in time to surface and manifest themselves in our lives, which will hinder the chance of our creating any positive experiences. But Virtue says, "If you tell yourself you've already accomplished a goal before you even start, you're way ahead of the game." In fact, just saying affirmations every day can make a tremendous difference in your life. According to psychotherapist and creator of guided-image audiotapes Belleruth Naparstek, we "don't have to believe in them [affirmations] for them to work." Author Susan Jeffers, Ph.D., explains that by saying something enough times, "it eventually becomes branded in your mind" (*Feel the Fear . . . and Beyond,* Ballantine, 1998).

I use a number of affirmations and healing words in my day-to-day life. I have collected uplifting quotations and poems for as long as I can remember. One of my personal favorites is by William Arthur Ward, and it hangs in my meditation room. It goes like this:

Choose not happiness, it will elude you
Pursue not pleasure, it will delude you
Trust not wealth, it will rule you
Follow not fame, it will fool you
Seek God's presence, it will bless you

You can choose any positive wording for your affirmations, like *peace, joy,* a line from a poem that speaks to you, and so forth. You can even make some up. Here are a few ideas to get you started:

- I am joyfully releasing anger and frustration.

- The more I pay attention to what I want, the quicker it becomes a reality in my life.

- I am blessed and whole.

- My support is eternal, and it comes from within.

- Everything in my life works out for the best, no matter what.

- I am enjoying every moment of my life.

- I feel safe with other people, and other people feel safe with me.

- God is love.

- I am loved.

- I am trusting the flow of life.

- I am taking responsibility and forgiving myself and others.

The Benefits of Affirmation

Raise your self-image and see the hidden worth of your life. Affirmations can help you:

- empower your attitude

- raise your self-esteem

- enhance your inner reality

- create positive changes in your life

Tips on Using Affirmations

There are a variety of ways to use affirmations. Here are a few that might work for you.

1. Look at yourself in the mirror and say out loud the affirmation you've chosen.

2. Study the words on a page.

3. Record yourself speaking the affirmation, then listen to it throughout the day.

4. Write the affirmation several times.

5. Say the affirmation you've chosen while doing your regular daily activities.

Getting your inner self in balance is critical in achieving living beauty and good health. It also creates a pathway where you can give yourself permission to soar through life with a newfound sense of freedom and explore the world of possibilities that are ready and waiting for you.

And once you've begun creating a more beautiful you through cleansing your inner environment, you'll be ready for the next step—detoxing your outer environment. And that is essential to your beauty goals since everywhere you look, your appearance is being thwarted on a regular basis. But don't despair! The next chapter is filled with helpful yet simple ways to further enhance your health and vivacious beauty by cleansing your home surroundings.

10

Detoxing the Outer

Life in all its fullness is Mother Nature obeyed.
WESTON A. PRICE

Beauty thieves are everywhere, especially in your home environment. They rob you of rejuvenating and cleansing vitamins, minerals, and enzymes as they creep into your body through food, air, and water. And since these beauty thieves can be absorbed through the skin, you need to pay closer attention these days to the cosmetics you're using as well as to the household chemicals surrounding you at home. Rashes, allergies, dermatitis, blotchy skin, blemishes, in addition to being health hazards, can all be linked to these xenoestrogenic beauty robbers. There is good news, however. Effective, nontoxic alternatives are available that are quite inexpensive. Plus, there are a number of easy ways to keep your indoors a haven, protecting your beauty and securing better health.

Cosmetics

The actual meaning of the word *cosmetic* is "to adorn." But the question is, with what? Synthetic, artificial, and even natural agents can all be potentially harmful to your body. The biggest problem that I've noticed with cosmetics today is that they often contain strong irritants. For instance, sodium lauryl sulfate, a powerful detergent agent found in shampoos, and even the essential oils lemon, ylang-ylang, sandalwood, and peppermint, can create sensitivities when applied directly to the skin. Some of these ingredients can even be downright toxic, adding another level of xenohormones to your system. As touched upon earlier in the book, cosmetics (like food) are often an overlooked source of the petrochemical xenohormones you need to avoid. These fat-soluble toxins enter your life in the form of coal tar dyes, emulsifiers, solvents, and artificial fragrances, and they accumulate over time. Plus, they gain immediate access to your body though the shampoo, makeup, hair dye, hair sprays, lipstick, and nail care products like fingernail polish and polish remover you use every day.

Now I'm not suggesting that you "go fanatic" or become neurotic over purchasing cosmetics. But it would be a good idea to avoid as much as possible products made with petrochemicals, such as mineral oil, petrolatum, synthetic colors, and synthetic fragrances. However, if you wish to take your cosmetic watch a step further, you may be quite interested in a report that came out several years ago, which brought the dangers of cosmetics to the public's attention. The *American Journal of Public Health* first reported in May 1988 that hair-dye use was linked to an elevated risk of leukemia and lymphoma, increasing with the extent of the exposure. That was the first bombshell. It was followed in July 1992 with a National Cancer Institute survey, also published in the *American Journal of Public Health*, which concluded that individuals who used hair dyes were far more likely to suffer from non-Hodgkin's lymphoma and multiple myeloma.

How do you know what to avoid? Aubrey Hampton, a pioneer in the field of natural, petrochemical-free cosmetics, has compiled a list entitled the "Ten Synthetic Cosmetic Ingredients to Avoid." By the way, some of his hair-care products are among my personal all-time favorites in the natural beauty arena. The following items are taken from Hampton's booklet, *Natural Ingredients Dictionary Plus Ten Synthetic Cosmetic Ingredients to Avoid,* listing known cosmetic irritants as well as petrochemicals:

1. Imidazolindyl Urea and Diazolindyl Urea. The most commonly used preservatives after the parabens. They are well established as a primary cause of contact dermatitis (American Academy of Dermatology). Two trade names for these chemicals are Germall II and Germall 115. Neither of the Germall chemicals has a good antifungal and must be combined with other preservatives. Germall 115 releases formaldehyde at just over 10 degrees. Both are considered toxic.

2. Methyl and Propyl and Butyl and Ethyl Paraben. Used as inhibitors or microbial growth and to extend shelf life of products. Widely used even though they are known to be toxic. Have caused many allergic reactions and skin rashes. Methyl paraben combines benzoic acid with the methyl group of chemicals. Highly toxic.

3. Petrolatum. This mineral oil and jelly causes a lot of problems when used on the skin. It can produce photosensitivity (promoting sun damage) and tends to interfere with the body's own natural moisturizing mechanism, leading to dry skin and chapping. Products containing petrolatum create the very conditions they claim to alleviate. Manufacturers use petrolatum because it is unbelievably cheap.

4. Propylene Glycol. Ideally it is a vegetable glycerin mixed with grain alcohol, both of which are natural. But usually it is a synthetic petrochemical mix used as a humectant. Has been known to cause allergic and toxic reactions.

5. PVP/VA Copolymer. A petroleum-derived chemical used in hair sprays, wave sets, and other cosmetics. It can be considered toxic, since particles may contribute to foreign bodies in the lungs of sensitive persons.

6. Sodium Lauryl Sulfate. This synthetic substance is used in shampoos for its foam-building abilities. It causes eye irritations, skin

rashes, hair loss, scalp scurf similar to dandruff, and allergic reactions. It is also frequently disguised in pseudonatural cosmetics with the parenthetic explanation "comes from coconut."

7. Stearalkonium Chloride. A chemical that causes allergic reactions and is used in hair conditioners and creams. Stearalkonium chloride was developed by the fabric industry as a fabric softener and is a lot cheaper and easier to use in hair conditioning formulas than proteins or herbals, which do help hair health. Toxic.

8. Synthetic Colors. The synthetic colors used to supposedly make a cosmetic "pretty" should be avoided at all costs, along with hair dyes. They will be labeled as FD&C or D&C followed by a color and a number. Example: FD&C Red No. 6 or D&C Green No. 6. Synthetic colors are believed to be cancer-causing agents. If a cosmetic has them in it, don't use the cosmetic.

9. Synthetic Fragrances. The synthetic fragrances used in cosmetics can have as many as two hundred ingredients. There is no way to know what the chemicals are because the label will simply say "fragrance." Some of the many problems caused by these chemicals are headaches, dizziness, rash, hyperpigmentation, violent coughing, vomiting, and skin irritation. Advice: Don't buy a cosmetic that has the word *fragrance* on the ingredients label.

10. Triethanolamine. Often used in cosmetics to adjust the pH. Also used with many fatty acids to convert acid to salt (stearate), which then becomes the base for a cleanser. TEA causes allergic reactions, including eye problems and dryness of hair and skin. It can also be toxic if absorbed into the body over a long period of time.

Your goal is to reduce toxic overload as much as possible. So if you would like to learn more about my own favorite kitchen cosmetic recipes—some of which are good enough to eat, the only gold standard for true "purity"—please refer to the "Natural Tips and Beauty Routines" section of chapter 8. By the way, a "natural" cosmetic is not necessarily a guarantee of purity; all you have to do is scan the ingredients of many health food store cosmetic lines to see what I mean.

Foods

Going organic is a sure way of decreasing your consumption of pesticides. But another reason to choose organic foods is that conventionally grown fruits and vegetables are severely lacking in beauty-specific nutrients that give you younger-looking skin, lustrous hair that is not graying and thinning, and strong bones, nails, and teeth. The fact is that just about every nutrient in our soil—and now, our produce—has sharply declined, as researcher Paul Bergner documented in his outstanding book, *The Healing Power of Minerals, Special Nutrients, and Trace Elements* (Prima, 1997). Bergner reports, for instance, that the amount of vitamin A—the skin vitamin par excellence—in some fruits (such as oranges, bananas, and apples) has dropped by approximately 66 percent since 1963. That means you would have to eat three pieces of these fruits to equal the vitamin level you would have received in just one piece three decades ago. Likewise, the amount of bone-building calcium in leafy green vegetables (like broccoli, romaine lettuce, iceberg lettuce, collard greens, Swiss chard) decreased on average by 46.4 percent. And studies of carrots, potatoes, tomatoes, corn, and celery demonstrate an average loss of 35 percent in cell-rebuilding magnesium content.

And pesticides, a well-recognized source of xenohormones, are now being connected to hormone-related disease from low sperm counts to breast cancer and immunosuppression. According to Charles Benbrook, a consultant to Consumer's Union, who was interviewed in the June 1997 *Nutrition Action Health Letter,* published by the Center for Science in the Public Interest: "We know that prolonged exposure to pesticides raises the risk of some cancers, neurological problems like Alzheimer's and Parkinson's diseases and developmental problems. It can also weaken the immune system, which leaves us more vulnerable to disease." Benbrook went on to say that pesticide exposure could impair, block, or disrupt both the development and the normal triggering of the immune system.

As discussed, secondhand hormones in conventionally raised beef and poultry as well as the bovine growth hormone known as rBGH in milk give you even more reasons to eat organic food. However, if you aren't already buying organic, you may want to start by purchasing pesticide-free poultry and beef from local farmers or a food co-op. (See the Resources section for suggestions.) While shopping at your favorite health food store or natural food co-op, you may want to buy organic dairy products and organic eggs as well.

Even if you've "gone organic," you may not realize that the most toxic foods around are ones you may still be ingesting: coffee and chocolate. Both coffee and chocolate are loaded with pesticides because many xenohormonic pesticides that are forbidden in this country are used in countries exporting their coffee and cocoa beans to us. For example, cocoa beans (used to make chocolate) are often dripping with pesticides like lindane, a pesticide the Environmental Protection Agency considers "probably carcinogenic." In Malaysia, one of the major countries exporting cocoa beans to us, the main sprayers of the cocoa beans are women, who know that the most popular way to commit suicide in their country is to drink the pesticides they are spraying on the cocoa beans. And so, if you are still addicted to chocolate, I urge you to at least search out brands that are certified organic. (See Resources for more help.)

Coffee lovers might look for certified organic coffee as well as the words *shade grown* on the label to ensure that the coffee beans didn't come in contact with the pesticides from the plantation-grown variety.

Fruits and Vegetables

You've read in past chapters about the importance of buying organic produce because some of our favorite fruits and vegetables contain major beauty-disrupting pesticides. The following chart appeared in the June 1997 issue of *Nutrition Action*, rating the most highly pesticide laden fruits and vegetables, both domestic and imported. The chart was prepared by the Environmental Working Group of Washington, D.C., using FDA data. According to their research, the top ten pesticide-ridden types of produce are:

1. strawberries

2. cherries (U.S.)

3. apples

4. cantaloupe (Mexico)

5. apricots

6. grapes (Chile)

7. blackberries

8. pears

9. raspberries

10. nectarines

According to this article, "the FDA detected a total of 30 different pesticides on different batches of strawberries. For example, 70 percent of all strawberries contained at least one pesticide and 36 percent contained two or more. Strawberries were also laced with the highest average levels of 'endocrine disrupters,' which can mimic or interfere with hormones."

So by all means, locate organic strawberries, cherries, and apples for your seasonal detox menus. I am quite serious when I say that the fate of our next generation may very well depend on our ability to limit as much as possible our exposure to petrochemical xenohormones. What better way then through life-sustaining beauty foods?

And remember, fruits and vegetables are not the only source of harmful pesticides. Like toxins, pesticides are often stored in an animal's body fat, where they accumulate over time into dangerous concentrations. In fact, some species of freshwater and saltwater fish these days contain a variety of toxins like the xenoestrogenic DDT, dioxin, PCBs, and heavy metals such as mercury. Since the toxins accumulate in the skin, organs, and fat of the fish, it's best to avoid eating the skin or excess fish fat in general. You'll still get your dose of omega-3s throughout the body of the fish. The FDA has recommended that we limit our intake of fish like orange roughy, grouper, and marlin to about two times per week because of the presence of mercury. Also pregnant women should probably eat high-mercury fish like swordfish or shark only once a month. You can always check the EPA's Web site for the latest advisories at www.epa.gov/ost/fish.

For nonorganic produce as well as commercial fish, eggs, and beef, consider the hydrogen peroxide soak discussed in chapter 3. And as a side note, because plastics are also a source of those nasty xenohormones, try not to heat your food in plastic or store it in plastic containers. Glass is my preference.

Water: The Chlorine Connection

Chlorine is another prevalent toxic chemical with xenohormonic properties. Used as a disinfectant against bacteria in drinking water, chlorine destroys the premier, rejuvenating antioxidant, vitamin E, which is crucial for feminine beauty, exquisite skin texture, and firm muscle tone. And chlorine has also been linked to heart disease as well as cancer. Even if you don't drink chlorinated water anymore, think of how many times you may swim, shower, or bathe in it. Chlorine, similar to other xenobiotics, can gain entrance into your body through the skin, most conveniently through your morning shower.

Chlorine reacts with water's natural organic matter creating new compounds called trihalomethanes, or THMs, which are carcinogenic. The best known and best researched of the THMs is chloroform. Chloroform is a solvent and a general anesthetic—the stuff used to knock people out—and can cause kidney, liver, and nervous system damage and has been associated with cancer in laboratory experiments. If there is chlorine in your water, you are being sprayed with chloroform every time you take a shower. Emissions from hot showers can dissolve 50 percent of the chlorine and 80 percent of other carcinogens like tetrachlorethylene and radon in the water. You are then breathing and soaking in these chemicals through your skin.

As you can see, drinking contaminated water is not the only way water becomes dangerous to your health. One-half of all water pollution exposure is through the skin and lungs via hot showers and baths. At the beginning of July 1997, the public health commissioner of Washington, D.C., issued a warning to the elderly, individuals with compromised immune systems, and the parents of infants to boil tap water before drinking it, according to Dr. Julian Whitaker in his newsletter, *Health & Healing*. Another news flash came just days later announcing that the city would add 60 percent more chlorine to its water supply. Oddly, officials stated that this high-level chlorinated water was safe for people to drink—they just shouldn't pour it into aquariums since it would kill fish!

Granted, chlorination is effective against many (but not all) bacteria in water. Experts, however, increasingly question the wisdom of trading the risk of bacterial infection for the risk of bladder cancer. Some are strongly against all chlorination of drinking water. Others suggest a change in its technology, including increased use of granular activated charcoal and the use of ozone gas. Plus, making chlorination the last rather than initial step of water treatment would reduce the amount of trihalomethanes.

How to Purify Your Water

Many individuals may be interested in a home water treatment system. My recommendation for home water treatment is a three-stage ceramic water filter, one of the most effective water filtration systems available. The filter is made of ultrafine ceramic with pores so small that they trap bacteria, parasites, and particles down to 0.5 microns in size. Unlike some other filter systems, this type doesn't create an environment for bacterial growth inside itself.

In the first stage, the tiny pores in the ceramic remove bacteria, parasites, rust, and dirt. The second filter stage is composed of high-density matrix carbon, which removes chlorine, pesticides, and other chemicals. And in the third stage, a special compound removes the heavy metals lead and copper.

One advantage of a three-stage ceramic water filter over the water distillation method is time—it can take up to six hours to distill a gallon of water using the latter method. This type of filter is also better than reverse osmosis because it doesn't waste water like the reverse osmosis method, which uses three gallons to produce one gallon of drinkable water. It also retains its maximum effectiveness for up to 1,100 gallons of water. So on average, a family of four would need to change the filter only once a year. The ceramic cartridge can be conveniently removed at any time for a light scrubbing.

If, however, nitrates or other heavy metals are present, a reverse osmosis system can be used in combination with a ceramic ultraviolet filter.

If your water is hard with calcium (not magnesium) deposits, you might also consider a magnetic water conditioning system, a salt-free solution to treating hard water for residential and commercial applications. Magnetic fluid treatment accomplishes many of the same benefits of traditional salt softening without the contaminating effluence produced by most salt softeners. These systems have proven effective by both university testing and thousands of satisfied customers. (See Resources.)

If you are still using tap water, use only the cold water for drinking and cooking. There is a greater probability that the hot water contains lead, asbestos, and other pollutants. Let the cold water tap run for a few minutes until it is as cold as it can get to flush out the pipes. The longer water sits in the pipes, the higher the lead content.

Household Chemicals

Household cleaning products are downright scary stuff. According to some expert estimates, every year Americans use up to twenty-five gallons of household cleaning products that contains a variety of toxic ingredients. Hazardous substances and petrochemicals lurk in your friendly scouring powder, dishwashing detergent, laundry soap, fabric softeners, and window cleaners. Only about two thousand of the chemicals in commercial use have been evaluated by the National Toxicology Program. At this time, nearly two hundred are considered carcinogenic.

Xenohormonic pesticides should be avoided and replaced with nontoxic alternatives. This pertains especially to lawn pesticides, garden pesticides, and ant, fly, and flea sprays. If you can't find a suitable substitute for your lawn and garden pesticides, then at least remember to wear gloves plus a protective mask, because harmful toxins can soak through your skin and lungs.

There are over fifty thousand pesticides available on the market, many of which are responsible for severe health problems. Perhaps the most toxic was a chemical used for termite control called chlordane, which remains toxic for up to twenty years. It can seep into 80 percent of all treated homes even when applied outside the home underground and has been linked to neurologic disorders, miscarriages, and cancers. Luckily in 1987 it was taken off the market, although exterminators can still legally use what is left in their reserves.

As a preventive measure against termites, keep all firewood at least thirty feet from the house. Investigate the noncarcinogenic termite control products called "permethrins" to replace toxic termidicides if you already have termite infestation.

To eradicate ants, keep in mind they hate mint. So you can chase them out by mixing 1 cup of water with 2 teaspoons of essential oil of peppermint. Spray wherever they enter the house on windowsills, cabinets, doorways, countertops, and along baseboards.

Cockroaches can be eliminated by mixing equal parts baking soda and powdered sugar. Spread this mixture where they seem to congregate and repeat at one- to two-week intervals until they are gone. Citrus oils repel flies. Try spraying the room with citrus-scented spray or scratch the skin of an orange and leave it out. Beetles that burrow in your grains can be eliminated quite nicely by placing a bay leaf in each container or, better still, storing your grains and flours in the fridge.

Potentially as harmful are commercial glass cleaners, laundry detergents, bathroom cleaners, and all-purpose cleaners. Windex, that favorite standby, contains the neurotoxin butyl cellosolve, a solvent and degreaser, which can be absorbed via the skin. The laundry detergents I grew up with such as Tide, Gain, Dash, and All, old familiar friends in the laundry room, are sources of sodium silicate, a chemical that can create eye and skin burning. Then there is another corrosive ingredient, sodium sulfate, which is a known respiratory irritant that is also found in common laundry powders.

I personally suggest locating a distributor who sells biodegradable cleaning products. I have used these products for over twenty years and have found them to be extremely effective and nontoxic. Long before it became fashionable, many companies touted their cleaning products as environmentally safe, biodegradable, and free of phosphates, chlorine, borates, or nitrates. I use a mixture of a concentrated biodegradable all-purpose cleanser (about ¼ teaspoon to 16 ounces of water) for all of my multipurpose cleansing needs, including window washing. I find that dust does not settle on those sprayed surfaces. Some companies have even stronger disinfecting products known to be effective against bacteria, fungi, and viruses, including salmonella, staph, strep, herpes simplex types I and II, and HIV, among others. Like the all-purpose concentrates, they must also be diluted. I think they make excellent bathroom disinfectants.

Of course, those of you who are more adventurous and creative may want to make your own danger-free detergents. Here is a basic multipurpose spray cleanser you may want to experiment with from *Natural Cleaning for Your Home: 95 Pure and Simple Recipes* (Lark Books, 1998):

1 cup liquid Castile soap

¼ teaspoon baking soda

¼ teaspoon tea tree extract (Melaleuca linarifloia)

2 tablespoons witch hazel extract

4 drops essential oil of choice (optional)—I suggest an aromatic one like vanilla

Mix the ingredients together in a spray bottle and shake gently. This effective cleaner works well on stoves, countertops, the outside of refrigerators and microwaves, and virtually any place you'd use a conventional spray. This handy homemade detergent has a shelf life of six months.

Of course, you can always use those tried-and-true standbys like vinegar, baking soda, and borax for nontoxic alternatives, when diluted with water in liquid or paste form.

Clear the air, but not with commercially produced air fresheners, which can be toxic and irritating. Instead, use alternatives such as fresh aromatic flowers. Aromatherapy essential oils like lavender, rosemary, and eucalyptus can be diffused to clean the air and clean your sinuses. Naturally, it's always a good idea to open windows, even in the middle of winter, for at least twenty minutes to clear the air. Also try common household plants, such as spider plants, elephant ear philodendron, Boston ferns, English

ivy, and aloe vera. More than decorative, they've been found by former
NASA scientist Bill Wolverton, Ph.D., to be effective in removing a wide
variety of indoor air pollutants. As Wolverton eloquently states in the
December 1997 *Townsend Letter for Doctors and Patients:*

> To the human eye, plants may appear static and nonreactive as
> they continue their normal process of living and growing. But in
> scientific terms, plants are highly dynamic, actively creating and
> emitting a cloud of complex, invisible substances around their
> leaves and roots that provide for their protection and well being.
> Houseplants do more than enhance the appearance of our sur-
> roundings: They can play an integral role in improving the very
> essence of our lives, the air we breathe.

Interiors

Use hardwood floors and glazed tiles in place of wall-to-wall carpeting
and linoleum. For the wood floors, use the best grade of thoroughly dried
solid oak without chemical sprays. If you must use carpeting, why not settle on some exquisite cotton area rugs or natural wool rugs rather than the
synthetics, which contain formaldehyde and other toxic chemicals? You
may not realize it, but carpeting is a surprisingly toxic source of indoor
pollution. It's heavily sprayed with insecticides, which can harbor molds,
mites, house dust, and noxious odors. Even so-called natural wool carpets
can be toxic because they may be moth proofed with chemicals. Another
problem with wall-to-wall carpet is the xenohormonic adhesives or glues
and solvents on the backing of the carpets, which can outgas for years at a
time, creating a steady stream of toxic emissions.

Similarly, choose furniture that is made of hardwood and untreated fabrics. Most furniture today is made from particleboard and/or veneered
wood, both of which are high in contaminants such as formaldehyde. You
can order furniture and fabrics from manufacturers that haven't been
treated with fire retardants and pesticides. The same is true of curtains
and drapes. Or you can use metallic miniblinds for window covering. Also,
natural cotton futons that haven't been chemically treated are good beds.

As you can imagine, you can become extremely overwhelmed, searching for chemical-free paints and varnishes. Look for paints that don't have mold inhibitors and preservatives. There are many natural paints and stains on the market today.

Creating a Relaxing Environment

Not only is it important to detox your outer environment, it is essential to create a state of calm in your home's interior. A good place to start is your bedroom, since we typically spend up to one-third of our lives in bed. This of all rooms in your home should exude a sense of harmony and relaxation and be a place you can retreat to for comfort when you're feeling down or ill. And as one of the more common lovemaking niches, the bedroom should be dedicated to warmth, giving, and privacy.

That's why it's important to make sure everything, from the carpeting to furniture, is constructed with healthy, not synthetic, materials. Exposure to these potentially destructive toxins night after night can undo the harmonic balance you've been trying so hard to create and can contribute to breathing problems, itchy eyes and skin, headaches, irritability, and fatigue. The culprits? Foam pillows and mattresses made of polyurethane or polyester; no-iron sheets having formaldehyde in their fabric; particleboard furniture that gives off chemical vapors; and paints and wallpapers made from petrochemicals. To lower possible allergic and toxic risks, start:

- using nonallergenic natural fabrics instead of synthetic ones

- replacing your sheets and pillowcases with 100 percent pure cotton or linen ones (cotton flannel is typically untreated)

- sleeping on a mattress that's made of natural fiber—latex foam is good

- purchasing blankets and quilts made of lamb's wool or cellular wool

Your beauty rest and health can also be disturbed, according to new data, by sleeping near electromagnetic fields (such as high-voltage power lines). In fact, electromagnetic radiation exposure has even been linked to cancer. Commonplace items in your bedroom may help increase this potential electromagnetic danger, from alarm clocks, TVs, and radios to lights near your bed, power sockets, and electric wiring. Also, bed frames made of steel or iron as well as spring mattresses, radiators, and plumbing equipment have the potential to become magnetic and disrupt the Earth's natural magnetic field. Removing these possible sources of health problems is vital, so here are some helpful tips:

- Move the position of your bed, keeping it away from electromagnetic objects.

- Keep in harmony with the Earth's magnetic field by sleeping in a north-south direction.

- Unplug all electrical items in your bedroom in the evening.

- Purchase battery-operated clocks, radios, and so forth.

Hopefully, you're becoming more enlightened about how vitality and living beauty depend upon removing toxins from your body and outer environment.

Now that your system is on its way to rejuvenation, energy, and healing, let's maintain that radiance by keeping an eye on telltale beauty signals and learning about all the beautifying nutrients that will replenish your body on a day-to-day basis.

11

Living Beauty Alphabet of Vitamins and Minerals

We're always the same age inside.
GERTRUDE STEIN

You possess the power to look your very best at every age and stage of life. Beautifying vitamins, minerals, and hormones create the gateway to clear, supple, skin, glorious-looking hair, and healthy nails. In fact, they are so fundamental to your appearance and well-being that many of these star nutrients are already built into the Living Beauty Detox Diet plan and seasonal maintenance tips. You'll also catch them playing major roles in the Natural Tips and Beauty Routines section outlined in chapter 8.

I'm a firm believer that the barrage of beauty problems plaguing many of us—like blotchy skin, splitting fingernails, lackluster hair, fatigue, stress, and weight gain—are actually secondary symptoms of vitamin, mineral, and other nutritional imbalances. As you have learned already, from the moment of birth, you began absorbing all sorts of unnatural and toxic substances from food, air, and the environment. And, as we've already discussed, your body was designed with a complex and sophisticated detoxification system, made up of the liver, skin, colon, kidneys, and lungs. These detoxification organs are capable of working with a precision not duplicated in any of our modern-day inventions.

Your skin, for instance, is the largest organ in your body and dedicated to protecting you from foreign elements inside and out. In fact, your body gets rid of approximately one-third of its impurities through the skin. In order to do its job, the skin has to maintain a continual state of regeneration. New cells are created at the bottom, or basal, layer and then force their way to the next layer, called the granular layer. Within four weeks of their birth, these new cells make their debut on the outside surface of your skin (called keratin) wrapped in a granular material. In time, this outside layer sheds, taking some waste material with it. But, as I've shared throughout this book, your detoxification pathways must not only eliminate the breakdown products that result from the normal, everyday metabolic wastes, but also rid your body of xenoestrogens, heavy metals, and toxic chemicals. Consequently, your liver, colon, and kidneys work overtime, causing your skin to often act as another route for elimination. And when waste materials are pushed through your pores, well, I don't have to tell you what that looks like.

Perhaps you can begin to understand why I insist that cleansing is truly the missing link to buoyant health and beauty. But see for yourself. Look at your skin, hair, nails, and even your tongue. Now looks at the chart below to better understand what kind of signals your body has been sending—and take heed.

Watch for Flashing Signs Up Ahead!

Skin Problems	What Your Skin May Be Screaming Out For
acne	zinc, vitamins B_6 and A, acidophilus, and essential fatty acids (EFAS)

Skin Problems, cont.	What Your Skin May Be Screaming Out For
pimples	chromium and a sugar-free diet
no elasticity	pantothenic acid or pantethine, grape seed extract, the amino acid proline
blackheads	vitamins A and B_6
eczema	a wheat- or dairy-free diet; vitamins A, C, and B complex, zinc, and EFAS
dry skin	vitamin A, vitamin E, and EFAS (flaxseed and evening primrose oil)
itchiness	more acid for the skin's natural acid mantle, and EFAS (flaxseed and evening primrose oil)
loss of skin pigmentation	B complex, especially PABA, folic acid, and B_{12}
brown spots or liver spots	antioxidants such as vitamins C and E and selenium; and superantioxidants like Pycnogenol® and grape seed extract, and glutathione
oily skin	B complex vitamins, especially B_6
wrinkles	protein and vitamin A
cracks around mouth	B complex vitamins, especially B_2
dull skin tone	detoxification
large pores	vitamins A and B complex
melasma (mask of pregnancy)	zinc and progesterone
broken capillaries	vitamin C and antioxidant bioflavonoids, such as Pycnogenol®, grape seed extract, and a copper-free diet
psoriasis	folic acid, vitamin B_{12}, EFAS, and detoxification
scars	vitamin E and sulphur
paleness	iron or folic acid and B_{12}
sunburn	EFAS and calcium
hives	EFAS and calcium
collagen loss	vitamin C and the amino acid proline
dark circles under eyes	detoxification and an allergy-free diet *Continued*

Skin Problems, cont.	What Your Skin May Be Screaming Out For
crow's feet	the antioxidant lutein
seborrheic dermatitis	B vitamins, especially B_6 and biotin; EFAS and zinc
facial hair	progesterone

Hair Problems	What Your Hair May Be Screaming Out For
dryness, split ends	EFAS
dandruff	vitamins A, B_6, B_{12}, and zinc
itchiness	more acid for the skin's natural acid mantle, EFAS, and vitamin E
hair loss	protein, B complex (especially biotin), and sulfur
dull, lifeless hair	vitamins A and E, choline, and EFAS
weak hair	zinc, silica, spring horsetail extracts
thinning hair	thyroid gland support, progesterone, protein, and zinc
slow hair growth	B complex, protein, and zinc
male-pattern baldness	standardized saw palmetto extracts
gray hair	PABA, inositol, choline, iron, copper, zinc, and trace minerals
chemotherapy-induced hair loss	vitamin C

Nail Problems	What Your Nails May Be Screaming Out For
ridges	detoxification or iron, calcium, vitamin A, and EFAS
brittle nails	EFAS, sulfur, vitamins A and B complex (especially biotin)
white spots	zinc
hangnails	B complex and vitamin C
fungus	detoxification from systemic yeast or Candida albicans
flattened nails	iron
concave, spoon-shaped	iron
nail-biting habit	calcium

Tongue Problems	What Your Tongue May Be Screaming Out For
magenta-colored tongue	vitamin B, especially B_2 (riboflavin)
fiery-red tongue or too large/small	vitamin B, especially B_3 (niacin)
beefy tongue	vitamin B, especially pantothenic acid
smooth at tip and sides; beefy, strawberry-red tongue	vitamin B, especially folic acid and B_{12}

A good deal of these beauty problems can be either eliminated or greatly reduced once you take action and incorporate the essential building blocks of beauty, which are listed below. These specific vitamins, minerals, EFAs, and hormones—which form the very fabric of beauty—can help you lay a strong foundation for good health and lifelong, radiant looks. So let's start to uncover *your* vibrant beauty by getting back to the basics, or rather the ABCs of beauty.

Beautifying Vitamins

Holding a prime role in affecting your appearance, vitamins are absolutely essential for creating new cells to keep your skin looking renewed. And, with their enzyme components, vitamins are helpful in regulating the metabolism of carbohydrates and fats, and support body tissues on a cellular level. Although vitamins are needed in relatively very small amounts, the body cannot manufacture most of them on its own. They must be obtained from food or through dietary supplements.

Vitamin A

The number one wrinkle fighter. By nurturing the fat lying beneath the skin, vitamin A, a fat-soluble vitamin, helps ensure skin that is taut, silky soft, and youthful looking. It also plays a role in absorbing the nucleic acid RNA, which further aids in retarding the aging process. If you lack sufficient amounts of this prime beauty vitamin, your appearance may suffer in a number of ways. For instance, your eyes may lose their gleam, you could develop night blindness, your nails may split, you might experience "bumpy, pimply" skin, your hair may become dry, and you could have problems with dandruff. Since vitamin A is fat soluble, your body can store it. Which means you must be cautious of elevated supplemental intakes, which lead to toxicity.

Beauty Foods Rich in Vitamin A: fish liver oils (especially shark and cod-liver oils), cantaloupe, pumpkin, sweet potato, carrots, mango, spinach, turnip greens, apricots, kale, parsley, collard greens, papaya, juice concentrate of kamut, barley, oat, and alfalfa grasses

Optimum Beauty Daily Dosage: 10,000–25,000 IUs, or up to 50,000 IUs (if under the care of a practitioner); if pregnant or trying to become pregnant, keep dosages to below 10,000 IUs.

Possible Beauty Overdose: over 25,000 IUs daily; or if pregnant, over 10,000 IUs daily

Vitamin B Complex

The nerve soother. In today's hectic world, B complex is essential in metabolizing sugar for energy and in relieving nervous tension and irritability, which wind up as stress lines on your face or contribute to ruining your posture. B vitamins also have a remarkable impact on your hair and skin: they give sheen to hair, help if you are losing hair or have premature graying, and assist in combating skin disorders like dermatitis. Menopausal women find extra benefit with these vital nutrients, which help lessen the troublesome ailments associated with this stage of life. Plus they're a good way to aid your liver in neutralizing any estrogen overload it may experience, per Guy Abraham, M.D. Sugar, alcohol, and coffee rob you of these critical water-soluble vitamins, which must be replaced daily. B vitamins work best when they're taken together. Some of the most critical to sustaining your beauty are discussed below.

Beauty Foods Rich in the Complete Vitamin B Family: organ meats (liver, brains, heart, kidney), oysters, cottage cheese, wheat germ, nutritional yeast, whole grains, soybeans, peas, watercress, asparagus, whey, red clover, oatstraw, parsley

Vitamin B_1 (Thiamin)

A helper in maintaining your weight, vitamin B_1 stabilizes appetite. It also acts as shield by cushioning the blow caused by everyday pressures. And that means you'll be wearing that brilliant smile of yours more often so your eyes and face radiate. As with all B vitamins, thiamin must be replaced each day. Note: alcohol use, sugar intake, smoking, and heat can all play a part in depleting your B_1 levels.

Beauty Foods Rich in Vitamin B_1: wheat germ, liver, whole grains and breads, nutritional yeast, salad greens, alfalfa, egg yolks, meat, oysters, nuts, sesame seeds, soybeans, blackstrap molasses, bran, lentils, oats, barley grass, spirulina, seaweeds

Recommended Beauty Daily Dosage: 10–500 mg.

Possible Beauty Overdose: none recognized

Vitamin B_2 (Riboflavin)

A protector, this beauty booster helps you have glistening eyes, calm nerves, strong nails, shiny hair, as well as a rosy glow, thanks to its aiding the hemoglobin in your blood. Since it is water soluble, you must maintain proper levels, otherwise thinning hair or hair loss, fissures around your mouth, whistle lines around the lips, scaly skin, oily skin, and whiteheads can mar your beauty. A deficiency could also cause your eyes to burn and become sensitive to light.

Beauty Foods Rich in Vitamin B_2: milk, meat, cottage cheese, yogurt, liver, eggs, green leafy vegetables, spirulina, chlorella, almonds, soybeans, nutritional yeast, avocados, peas, fenugreek, rose hips, nettles

Recommended Beauty Daily Dosage: 10–50 mg.

Possible Beauty Overdose: above 50 mg. has been linked to cataract formation

Vitamin B_6 (Pyridoxine)

This vitamin is so beneficial to female needs that it's often regarded as a guardian angel to women. It's an antidermatitis nutrient, often used to treat troubled skin, including acne, dry scalp, oily skin, thinning hair, hair loss, dandruff, dermatitis, and stretch marks. And since vitamin B_6 is key in metabolizing fatty acids and fats, you enjoy a more youthful, healthy-looking skin. It acts as a cofactor with essential fatty acids to put a sheen in your hair. For menstruating women—typically teens, twenties, thirties, forties—B_6 is a principal player in lessening PMS symptoms such as bloating, blemishes, mood swings, depression, and anxiety. It's also a big hit for postmenopausal women since the vitamin performs multiple tasks like aiding in collagen formation and strengthening bones. As do other B vitamins, it takes the edge off nerves and supports your beauty rest.

Beauty Foods Rich in Vitamin B_6: liver, meat, fish, poultry, legumes, nutritional yeast, wheat germ, whole grains and breads, brown rice, soybeans, lentils, alfalfa, kale, spinach, bananas, nuts, egg yolks, milk, green vegetables, unsulphured molasses, bran

Recommended Beauty Daily Dosage: 10–200 mg.; pregnant women or those on the Pill require extra amounts to help with water retention and PMS tensions.

Possible Beauty Overdose: 500 mg. to 2 grams daily have been associated with severe motor and sensory neuropathies.

Vitamin B_{12}

Great for putting the zest back in your life, vitamin B_{12} helps you have a better frame of mind and overall improved well-being. It's particularly helpful for menopausal women, who often need a lift. Since it is vital for supporting red blood cells, it is also great for younger women concerned with anemia. It is also helpful for depression and memory loss. A sore, unusually red tongue, as well as fatigue, may signal a vitamin B_{12} deficiency. If you are a vegan, you'll need to take special care to secure proper amounts.

Beauty Foods Rich in Vitamin B_{12}: muscle meats, liver, fish (sardines, clams, salmon, flounder, lobster), poultry, kidney, eggs, yogurt, sea vegetables, spirulina

Recommended Beauty Daily Dosage: 50–5,000 mcg.

Possible Beauty Overdose: none recognized

Niacinamide (Niacin)

Absolutely required for healthful beauty throughout your life, niacin goes to work helping you radiate clear skin, healthy-looking gums for that winning smile, and improved circulation for a rosy glow. Recognized as good for lowering cholesterol, niacin also plays an important part in the metabolic breakdown of proteins, carbohydrates, and fats so your system attains all the beauty benefits of food nutrients. Although niacinamide does not reduce cholesterol levels or enhance circulation, it has proved to be helpful in treating osteoarthritis, especially important to postmenopausal women. Additionally, it has also been linked to the reduction of diabetic cases, according to a New Zealand study. If your system lacks sufficient amounts of this vital B vitamin (niacinamide/niacin), you could experience severe blemished skin known as pellagra, dermatitis, bad breath, depression, and even headaches.

Beauty Foods Rich in Niacin: nutritional yeast, fish (salmon, tuna), liver, heart, wheat germ, lean meat, poultry, peanuts, seeds, whole grains and breads, brown rice, alfalfa, wheat bran, spirulina, hops, licorice, nettles, parsley

Recommended Beauty Daily Dosage: of Niacin: 10–50 mg.; of niacinamide: 10–4,000 mg.

Possible Beauty Overdose: more than 35 mg. of niacin daily can cause itching and flushing; doses over 1,000 mg. a day could damage the liver.

PABA

This "vitamin inside of a vitamin" has been recognized for its antioxidant abilities, helping to prevent aging and maintaining the color and tone of the complexion. Because PABA helps activate folic acid production in the intestine, it also encourages pantothenic acid, vital for combating wrinkles and stress. In fact, it's used by doctors along with pantothenic acid and folic acid to bring back the color to graying hair, if stress or poor nutrition caused it. PABA is also a natural sunscreen, which makes it ideal for many cosmetic formulations, such as creams and suntan lotions. Lacking sufficient amounts of PABA—sulfa drugs contribute to a deficiency—could make you irritable, depressed, tired, and nervous. Your hair might also turn gray, and you could develop white patches on your skin.

Beauty Foods Rich in PABA: organ meats (liver, kidney, heart), nutritional yeast, fish, fruits, nuts, whole grains, sunflower seeds

Recommended Beauty Daily Dosage: 50 mg.

Possible Beauty Overdose: none recognized

Inositol

Your hair gets its sheen and fullness from this B vitamin. Inositol aids in emulsifying fats to fatty acids to support supple, firm skin and body form, puts a halt to cellulite, reduces plaque in your arteries, and aids in proper absorption of vitamin E. If you don't get enough of this extraordinary vitamin, your hair could start to thin and your skin could break out. Constipation, mood swings, irritability, and arteriosclerosis are also signs of an inositol deficiency, as is anxiety in sensitive individuals.

Beauty Foods Rich in Inositol: nutritional yeast, wheat germ, whole grains, fruits, organ meats, chickpeas (garbanzos), soy lecithin, lentils, barley, oats, beef, alfalfa, blackstrap molasses

Recommended Beauty Daily Dosage: 500–1,000 mg.

Possible Beauty Overdose: none recognized

Choline

Like inositol, the B vitamin choline also assists in the breakdown of fat and cholesterol to support soft skin and lustrous hair. Choline is also a tremendous aid in encouraging memory and nerve-impulse transmission as well as hormone production. In fact, neither your memory nor your brain function properly without it. Stunted growth, a compromised liver and kidney, gastric ulcers, and high blood pressures are some of the signs of a choline deficiency.

Beauty Foods Rich in Choline: organ meats, seeds, egg yolk, nutritional yeast, peanuts, wheat germ, corn germ, green leafy vegetables, lentils, split peas, brown rice, cabbage, soy lecithin

Recommended Beauty Daily Dosage: 500–1,000 mg.

Possible Beauty Overdose: In amounts of 3,500 mg. (3.5 grams) daily, vomiting, excessive sweating, and gastrointestinal upset have been reported.

Biotin

Proper biotin levels aid a smooth, clear complexion, gleaming eyes, vibrant hair, and properly functioning glands. Biotin also helps avert dermatitis, baldness, and weak nails. Plus, it's needed for your body to use protein, folic acid, B_{12}, and pantothenic acid. If you lack adequate amounts of biotin, you may have yeast infections, insomnia, muscle aches and pains, colorless skin, and even lesions on your skin. Eating raw egg yolks impedes absorption.

Beauty Foods Rich in Biotin: nutritional yeast, wheat germ, liver, cooked egg yolks, peanuts, whole brown rice, soybeans, split peas, lentils, green peas, tuna, sardines

Recommended Beauty Daily Dosage: 2–5 mg. for maximum beauty

Possible Beauty Overdose: none recognized

Folic Acid

A nutrient essential for energy, immune system support, and red blood cell formation, folic acid is invaluable to women. It contributes to your having healthy-looking skin, hair, and nails by aiding in protein metabolism. Plus, folic acid has been known to help alleviate anxiety and depression, which cause a tense or haggard look on your face. It is extremely important to women in their childbearing years. Folic acid has been connected to the prevention of birth defects such as spina bifida and anencephaly. It further aids in fetal development by regulating embryonic and nerve cell formations. Ideally, this star nutrient should be taken months prior to conception for optimal effect. So if you're trying to get pregnant, or even if you're already pregnant, folic acid should be part of your nutrient regimen. And doctors like Dr. Robert Atkins use folic acid as a natural form of hormonal replacement for perimenopausal and menopausal women.

Beauty Foods Rich in Folic Acid: kale, chard, spinach, asparagus, broccoli, beets, whole grains

Recommended Beauty Daily Dosage: Take 400–800 mcg. with vitamin B_{12} and vitamin C. If you want to get pregnant, take at least 800 mcg. Menopausal women, under a physician's care, can take megadoses of folic acid (20–40 mg.) as a natural estrogen replacement therapy. Since high amounts of folic acid can mask a B_{12} deficiency causing brain damage, do not increase supplementation unless you check with your nutritionally oriented physician.

Possible Beauty Overdose: none recognized

Pantothenic Acid

This important vitamin is critical for stopping wrinkles and premature aging in their tracks. Pantothenic acid encourages your body's production of cortisone as well as other vital hormones to give you silky skin. In addition, it helps give you adrenal support so you can fight stress. Consequently, a deficiency leads to adrenal burnout and troubled skin.

Beauty Foods Rich in Pantothenic Acid: muscle meats, liver, sardines, clams, salmon, flounder, lobster, poultry, kidney, egg yolk, yogurt, sea vegetables, spirulina

Recommended Beauty Daily Dosage: 25–1,000 mg.

Possible Beauty Overdose: In amounts of 10,000 mg. (10 grams) per day, water retention and diarrhea have been reported.

Vitamin C

Vitamin C is the wrinkle-fighting antioxidant critical for beautiful teeth, healthy-looking gums, strong capillary walls, and a functionally healthy immune system to ward off colds, allergies, and infections. It's also vital in supporting your connective tissue to guarantee you limber, yet elegant, movement. With special help from bioflavonoids, vitamin C helps build collagen, that gluelike compound needed in connective tissue for you to stay young looking. This antiaging vitamin also helps combat stress and varicose veins. Your body can't store it, so you'll need to get your daily dose of this magnificent beauty promoter. Available in either topical or supplement form.

Beauty Foods Rich in Vitamin C: rose hips, oranges, limes, lemons, kiwi, grapefruits, acerola cherries, black currants, strawberries, guava, papaya, mangoes, cantaloupe, pineapple, avocados, tomatoes, green peppers, bean sprouts, green leafy vegetables, parsley, green peppers, cabbage, dandelion greens, nettles, alfalfa, cayenne

Recommended Beauty Daily Dosage: 500–5,000 mg.

Possible Beauty Overdose: diarrhea can result from higher dosages

Vitamin D

You've already read how primary the sunshine vitamin D is for women. Thanks to its help, you'll enjoy lower blood pressure, strong bones, beautiful teeth, and better posture for a more graceful you. Getting fifteen minutes of vitamin D–rich sunlight daily will help your body use calcium. A vitamin D deficiency creates soft bones and subsequent dental troubles, so it is critical for postmenopausal women and those with osteoporosis. It is a fat-soluble vitamin that some researchers consider a hormone—that's how far-reaching its effects are.

Beauty Foods Rich in Vitamin D: butter, egg yolk, dairy products, nutritional yeast, tuna fish, herring, mackerel, salmon, sardines, shrimp, cod-liver oil

Recommended Beauty Daily Dosage: 400–800 IUs or sunlight. Postmenopausal women should take 600–800 IUs daily to protect against and help control osteoporosis.

Possible Beauty Overdose: none recognized

Vitamin E

Molecularly structured like estrogen, vitamin E can be helpful as a natural hormone replacement. It holds key positions in promoting good-looking skin, better health for your heart, and enhanced well-being. Vitamin E is a tremendous help to PMS sufferers when taken in conjunction with a B complex. And perimenopausal women gain relief from hot flashes, tender breasts, and vaginal dryness. Women going through menopause may also alleviate their irritating symptoms by taking this incredibly helpful vitamin. A lack of vitamin E produces an increased risk of infections, varicose veins, and dry, itchy skin. It is probably the most challenging vitamin to obtain through diet alone because even the richest beauty food sources fall short of the recommended dosage.

Beauty Foods Rich in Vitamin E: fresh unprocessed vegetable oils, fresh nuts, seeds, wheat germ, rose hips, dandelion

Recommended Beauty Daily Dosage: 100–1,200 IUs; if you have high blood pressure or are taking blood thinners (anticoagulant medication), start with 100 IUs and consult your doctor.

Possible Beauty Overdose: none recognized

Vitamin K

Produced in your intestines by healthy, friendly flora, vitamin K helps the liver do its job and contributes to the blood-clotting process. It is now emerging as a primary factor in bone mineral density and osteoporosis prevention. Radiation, rancid fats, antibiotics, and aspirin all deplete your body's levels of this valuable vitamin. Natural vitamin K supplements do not exist, so you may want to include yogurt and kefir in your diet since vitamin K is produced in an intestinal flora environment.

Beauty Foods Rich in Vitamin K: yogurt, kefir, cabbage, cauliflower, all leafy green vegetables, alfalfa, nettles

Recommended Beauty Daily Dosage: 150 mcg.; if you are taking blood thinners (anticoagulant medication), check with your physician before supplementing with vitamin K–rich foods.

Possible Beauty Overdose: none recognized

Beautifying Minerals

Vital for lifelong health, glowing complexion, resilient hair, strong teeth, and overall vibrant beauty, minerals renew and rejuvenate you. Minerals are the real beauty spark plugs because they function as coenzymes enabling vitamins and nutrients to produce energy and facilitate healing. Since they are dependent on one another, if one mineral is out of balance, all are affected. Ratios are key when it comes to minerals and their beauty benefits. Diuretics such as tea and coffee as well as higher-than-normal perspiration and/or urination can deplete many of the minerals critical to your appearance and health.

Calcium

Well known for its role in building strong teeth and bones as well as its fight against osteoporosis, calcium is paramount in the entire life cycle of a woman. It plays a critical role in muscular contractions and is regarded as a menstrual cramp inhibitor. It's also vital for perimenopausal insomnia and postmenopausal bone thinning. Calcium also keeps your heart beating in rhythm and can lower blood pressure and reduce colon cancer risk. However, as noted earlier in this book, calcium absolutely must be balanced with magnesium for proper absorption and complete value. The ratio should be 2:1 in favor of magnesium, the number one key to proper calcium absorption and building strong, flexible, healthy bones. Calcium is particularly important for women in their bone-building years (teens and twenties). Women in their thirties, forties, fifties, and above should be getting at least 500 mg., balancing their intake with the essential 2:1 magnesium-to-calcium ratio mentioned earlier. The most absorbable forms of calcium include calcium citrate, calcium aspartate, and chelated calcium. Sugar, alcohol, carbonated beverages, and caffeine all impede calcium absorption.

Beauty Foods Rich in Calcium: yogurt, cheese, milk, buttermilk, sardines, salmon, sesame seeds, turnip greens, cauliflower, blackstrap molasses, sea vegetables, bok choy, parsley, carrots, spinach, lentils, dandelions, nettles, peppermint, and oatstraw

Recommended Beauty Daily Dosage: 500–1,500 mg. in balance with other minerals and vitamins. The National Institutes of Health recommends that women twenty-five to fifty years old get 1,000 mg. per day. Pregnant or lactating women and postmenopausal women receiving estrogen replacement therapy—1,200 mg. per day; and postmenopausal women not receiving estrogen replacement therapy—1,500 mg. per day.

Possible Beauty Overdose: should be kept in 2:1 magnesium-to-calcium ratio

Magnesium

The star player in women's health, magnesium helps to balance and complement calcium in its function as a bone builder. It's extremely important that women suffering from PMS or those in the perimenopausal years adhere to a recommended 2:1 ratio of magnesium to calcium. Magnesium also holds a key place in rebuilding cells to ensure the most youthful appearance possible because it provides for flexible bones and arteries. Plus, it contributes to showing off your pearly whites by playing a critical part in building tooth enamel. When you are magnesium deficient, depression, that rundown feeling, fatigue, irritability, anxiety, nervous tension, and spasms result. If you're still menstruating and suffering from perimenopausal symptoms, magnesium helps combat nervousness and low blood sugar levels. It is also a must for younger women with PMS who suffer from cramps and menstrual-related migraine headaches. Alcohol, too much protein, birth control pills, menstruation, and synthetic vitamin D hamper magnesium absorption.

Beauty Foods Rich in Magnesium: almonds, leafy green vegetables, wheat germ, sea vegetables, blackstrap molasses, sunflower seeds, soybeans, lecithin, whole brown rice, corn, nettles, burdock, horsetail, evening primrose

Recommended Beauty Daily Dosage: 400–800 mg.

Possible Beauty Overdose: 600–800 mg. can make for loose stools, so just cut back to bowel tolerance.

Phosphorus

As the second most abundant mineral in your body, phosphorus and its co-workers, magnesium and calcium, help protect your teeth, skin, hair, and bones. It also helps calm your nerves and heighten the mental process, both so vital in our nonstop world. Watch out for sugar, which can thwart the calcium-phosphorous balance. A deficiency creates fatigue, irritability, anxiety, pains in your bones, weight fluctuations, and weakness.

Beauty Foods Rich in Phosphorus: red meat, sardines, wheat germ, almonds, pumpkin seeds, sesame seeds

Recommended Beauty Daily Dosage: 800 mg.; pregnant or lactating women should take up to 1,200 mg.

Possible Beauty Overdose: none recognized; however, high levels of phosphorus can upset the calcium balance and result in bone weakening.

Zinc

You've learned about this all-star beauty mineral already and its role in strong nails, vibrant hair, and supple skin. Zinc helps retard aging and aids in the absorption of many other vitamins and minerals. It is a must in the formation of collagen. Typically, younger women (in their teens and twenties) suffer from a zinc deficiency, which results in PMS problems like blood sugar imbalances and sugar cravings. And since it supports vitamin D functions, zinc plays a part in halting osteoporosis and proves valuable to menopausal women. Plus, it helps with adult-onset diabetes, commonly occurring during menopause. If you lack this trace mineral, your hair will not grow and it could become weak with split ends. Birth control pills, high copper levels in tissues from the copper IUD, copper water pipes, estrogen replacement therapy, and excessive alcohol consumption impede absorption.

Beauty Foods Rich in Zinc: red meat, eggs, pumpkin seeds, herring, oysters, whole grains, blackstrap molasses, whole bran, whole oatmeal, wheat germ, chicken, liver, sesame seeds, spirulina, sage, wild yam, nettles, and milk thistle

Recommended Beauty Daily Dosage: 15–30 mg. (zinc picolinate); if pregnant, 10–60 mg. Maintain a 10:1 ratio with copper.

Possible Beauty Overdose: more than 60 mg. daily may affect the cardiovascular system by lowering HDL (good cholesterol) levels.

Selenium

A super antioxidant that works synergistically with vitamin E, selenium stops free-radical production and, subsequently, supports your immune system. Plus, selenium halts inflammation and aids in removing toxins. It also helps give your tissues elasticity and helps to ensure proper functioning in your pancreas, liver, and heart. A selenium deficiency produces brittle nails, hair loss, garlic-smelling breath, blemishes, pale or yellowish skin, gastro problems, and arthritis.

Beauty Foods Rich in Selenium: beef, turkey, veal, eggs, whole cereal grains, Brazil nuts, cashews, broccoli, brown rice, garlic, kelp, coconut, mushrooms, fenugreek, black cohosh, hawthorn berries, rose hips

Recommended Beauty Daily Dosage: 100–200 mcg.

Possible Beauty Overdose: over 700 mcg. daily can contribute to bone thinning.

Sulfur

This beauty mineral—housed in every cell of your body—helps give sheen and gloss to your hair and strength to your nails. It is a vital part of protein molecules and with the B-complex vitamins plays an important role in building tissue and enhancing the health of your cells.

Beauty Foods Rich in Sulfur: broccoli sprouts, peanut butter, wheat germ, eggs, lentils, cheese, beef, clams, garlic, onions, green peppers, brussels sprouts, cabbage, asparagus, fish, legumes, sage, nettles, horsetail

Recommended Beauty Daily Dosage: 500 mg.

Possible Beauty Overdose: none recognized

Iron

Truly, iron is a double-edged sword. It can be good for menstruating women who lose iron-rich blood every month, resulting in potential anemia and its accompanying fatigue, lifeless hair, coldness, pale and dry skin, and dark circles under the eyes. Iron needs increase if you become pregnant, are nursing, or are indulging in heavy exercise. On the positive side, iron attaches to other vitamins to enhance your body's process. For instance, it works with vitamin A to protect your eyes, with vitamin C (which also increases iron absorption) to nurture connective tissue, and with the B vitamins for supple skin and shiny hair. It also helps manufacture red blood cells, which are vital to your oxygen supply and increase your energy and vitality.

But if you're not anemic or menstruating, iron supplementation can be downright dangerous, causing hemochromatosis, or iron overload. This condition affects 1 out of 300 Americans. As a matter of fact, an iron overload can actually speed up the aging process, up your chances of developing heart disease, and contribute to the production of free radicals that promote cancer cells. This is especially important for postmenopausal women who are no longer losing iron-rich blood every month and may start to store iron instead. However, women of all ages need to have a test to measure stored-iron levels—called a serum ferritin test—prior to adding iron to their diets. Until this test is done, taking an iron-free supplement is wise.

Beauty Foods Rich in Iron: dark green leafy vegetables, barley grass, spinach, beans, beets, unsulphured molasses, wheat germ, liver, red meat, oysters, grapes, avocados, raisins, apricots, seaweeds, kelp, egg yolk, pumpkin seeds, dandelion root, nettles, fenugreek, peppermint, burdock

Recommended Beauty Daily Dosage: if needed, typically 15 mg. for menstruating or lactating women; for those who are pregnant, 30 mg. Menopausal and postmenopausal women should opt for iron-free multivitamins unless a ferritin test is performed that shows low iron stores. In this case, women fifty and above can safely supplement with 10 mg. daily. (Iron glycinate and liquid liver extracts do not cause constipation like other iron preparations.)

Possible Beauty Overdose: any level, if you suffer from an iron overload

Copper

Much like iron, copper is another double-edged sword. You've read earlier about the downside of copper overload. However, in balance, copper does a great deal to enhance your beauty. It is intricately involved in regenerating cells, and it works with vitamin C to produce collagen and elastin, giving you youthful skin and a renewed appearance. In fact, copper peptide has been shown to provoke dermal collagen, which slows down your skin's aging process while increasing dermal moisture retention. Copper peptide also stimulates superoxide dismutase (SOD), a naturally occurring antioxidant enzyme, to fight those ugly free radicals that are out to ravage your looks and cause you to age prematurely. It also acts as a turbocharge, aiding your body's use of the biochemical energy in new tissues, like your skin. Subsequently, your skin creates a special substance called glycosuminoglycans (GAG) to retain moisture in its inner cells, plumping them up. Plus, copper peptide is critical for hair growth, for skin elasticity and firmness, and for healing wounds and torn tissues. You don't need all that much copper to get the many beauty benefits it offers. Remember, zinc must outrank copper in a 10:1 ratio. Constant stress, birth control pills, and estrogen dominance can all lead to an increase in copper.

Beauty Foods Rich in Copper: soy foods, chocolate, carob, regular tea, seafood, mushrooms, blackstrap molasses, wheat germ, sage, chickweed, skullcap

Recommended Beauty Daily Dosage: be tested first; a tissue mineral analysis or hair analysis is the most convenient and inexpensive way to determine a copper overload. If needed, 1–3 mg. This should be kept in a 10:1 zinc to copper ratio.

Possible Beauty Overdose: any level if you suffer from a copper overload

Manganese

Good for its antioxidant protection, manganese is a trace mineral that helps offset the destructive results of an iron overload. It's critical for your adrenal glands to work well, particularly during times of increased stress. Manganese also assists in hormone and enzyme functions that play a part in giving you a younger-looking visage. In addition, it helps with thyroid, brain, and sugar metabolism, making it a must for diabetics.

Beauty Foods Rich in Manganese: pumpkin seeds, nuts, eggs, lean beef, sea vegetables, whole grain cereals, beets, green vegetables, dandelion, milk thistle, hops, raspberry leaf

Recommended Beauty Daily Dosage: 10–30 mg.

Possible Beauty Overdose: over 30 mg., use with supervision, as manganese can build up in the system, resulting in certain types of mental disorders.

Beautifying EFAs

If you want to stop fine lines from appearing, then essential fatty acids are the key. They are invaluable to your skin, helping lubricate the fatty layer just beneath your skin. Besides giving you a dewy complexion everyone will admire, EFAs should be your constant companions since they provide sheen for your hair and softness to your skin as well as enhance the health of your arteries. Without EFAs, you may experience hair thinning or loss, dandruff, splitting nails, scaly skin, and dull hair. The most important thing to do is toss out those processed vegetable oils and hydrogenated fats (like margarine and vegetable shortening) you've been using and add flaxseed oil, virgin olive oil, or sesame oil to your menu, as suggested in the Living Beauty Detox Diet and maintenance plan. The essential fatty acid GLA has a tremendous impact on your skin by upping your body's energy production and creating more cell resilience. Consequently, you feel and look refreshed. A number of factors lessen the amount of GLA in your body, such as aging, hydrogenated fats, fried foods, sugar, thyroid malfunction, and low levels of magnesium, zinc, and vitamins C, B_3, and B_6.

Beauty Foods Rich in EFAs: golden unprocessed vegetable oils, flaxseed oil, fish oils, cold-water fish, salmon, sardines, mackerel, primrose oil, black currant seed, borage oil

Recommended Beauty Daily Dosage: 1–2 tablespoons of flaxseed oil; 500 mg. of GLA; 1,000–3,000 mg. of EPA (the omega-3 fatty acid found in fish oils)

Possible Beauty Overdose: none recognized, but be aware that fish oils can act as blood thinners and may be contraindicated if already taking blood-thinning medication.

Beautifying Hormones

Your sex hormones affect every part of your well-being, from your heart, brain, and bone health to your stress-coping mechanisms, immune system, and aging process. Designed to work together in harmony, these mystifying hormones also are vitally linked to your beauty.

Estrogen

Rather than a single substance, estrogen is a hormonal group composed of estradiol, estrone, and estriol. Depending on which stage of life you're in, one of these three plays a key role. For example, estradiol is an estrogen workhorse manufactured in the ovaries during your menstruating years. If you become pregnant, estriol is predominant. But once you become postmenopausal, estrone levels escalate. Overall, estrogen is a tough antioxidant that fights off those precarious free radicals trying to destroy your tissues. It also contributes to that rosy, vibrant glow you want by guarding arterial linings so blood can move along without being impeded. Plus, estrogen helps lower LDL and raise HDL cholesterol levels. Estrogen also aids in collagen production to keep your skin firm and toned as it supports hyaluronic acid production for moisture-rich skin. Besides giving your bladder tissues elasticity, estrogen has receptors in your bone to enhance your body's use of calcium and to reduce loose teeth, cavities, and soft bones. Based on salivary hormone levels, estrogen should be in a 200:1 ratio in favor of progesterone. Your estriol levels should be more dominant, typically in an 8:1 ratio over the other two estrogens.

Recommended Beauty Daily Dosage: evaluate your estrogen level first by using a salivary hormone test that evaluates proper levels and ratios by age (see Resources Section under Uni Key).

Possible Beauty Overdose: unopposed estrogen is connected to irritability, anxiety, hair loss, weight gain, and breast cancer.

Progesterone

You've already read a lot about how progesterone can help balance out estrogen dominance. Which is why keeping progesterone in a 200:1 ratio with estrogen is so vital. Progesterone is also a wonderful mood lifter and antidepressant. When you have a balance of progesterone in your system, you should have a sense of tranquillity and experience less anger and irritability, so common with excessive amounts of estrogen. Progesterone is the master controller, blocking receptors to ward off the excesses of another hormone. It also contributes to activating osteoblasts, those bone builders critical for a strong stature and graceful appearance. If your progesterone levels are too low, PMS symptoms can manifest, such as depression, irritability, weight gain, and food cravings. If you're menopausal and have decreased progesterone, your symptoms will typically escalate, resulting in sleeplessness, night sweats, low libido, and anxiety.

Recommended Beauty Daily Dosage: 20 mg. per day for topical progesterone creams; 100–200 mg. daily of oral, micronized progesterone

Possible Beauty Overdose: none recognized

Testosterone

Known for its libido-enhancing qualities, testosterone can greatly affect your beauty and general health. It's an anabolic hormone, which means it helps restore or build your body back up—essential after exercise or stressful situations. It also helps build strong muscles and ligaments to keep your body looking trim and firm. However, when menopause arrives, testosterone may lower by half or more. That's when tiredness, anxiety, depression, joint aches or pains, delicate dry skin, weight and muscle loss, osteoporosis, and low libido appear. If a menopausal women adds testosterone to her supplementation, she may very well begin to feel invigorated, regaining her energy and sexual drive.

Recommended Beauty Daily Dosage: determine your individual needs at your age and stage of life by using a salivary hormone test (see Resources section under Uni Key).

Possible Beauty Overdose: excessive amounts of testosterone have been linked to male characteristics such as voice deepening and excessive growth of hair on the face and body.

Your complete beauty alphabet will help you sustain a strong foundation that should last a lifetime. A French poet once wrote, "Every age has its pleasures, its style of wit, and its own ways." But the good news for all of us in the twenty-first century is that no matter what our biological age, we can rejuvenate and regenerate our beauty—in body and spirit—from the inside out. Cleansing is the secret key to beauty, to anti-aging, and to overall health. Learning how to cleanse in harmony with the seasonal cycles of Mother Nature will ensure that we feel vitally alive 365 days of the year. Staying beautiful (and healthy) in a toxic world may be a challenge, but truly, the future of our next generations depends on it.

H-3 Plus

The most exciting news I can leave you with is this: I have rediscovered what may be the single most important vitamin complex for health, beauty, and sustained energy. It is called H-3 Plus and is based upon the legendary Roumanian formula containing procaine, a potent anti-aging factor supported by over 300 clinical studies and thousands of testimonials. People all over the world are proclaiming relief of depression, arthritis, and fatigue, as well as increased energy, sex drive, hair regrowth, and the return of their original hair color and texture.

H-3 Plus is protected by four unique U.S. patents. It can be purchased by my readers through Uni Key (see Resources). Won't you join me in the Living Beauty crusade?

Appendix: The Two-Week Fat Flush

The human body has one ability not possessed
by any machine—the ability to repair itself.
GEORGE E. KIRLEY JR., M.D.

The Two-Week Fat Flush is a quick way to cleanse the accumulated bad fats in the tissues and liver. It also prevents new fats, in the form of triglycerides, from forming and reestablishes a beneficial fat ratio in the brown fat tissues for continued weight stabilization, fat-burning stimulation, and appetite control.

Some people lose up to ten inches at the waist, buttocks, and thighs, whereas they may lose only five pounds on the scale. This two-week plan flushes out fat that normal diets don't. On this program, you will lose weight and begin to metabolize the toxic water and fat accumulation in your body.

If you are doing the program mainly for weight loss, weigh yourself only once a week. People do not lose weight at the same rate, and you can get discouraged if you hit a plateau. You can completely redistribute your weight on this program without a dramatic loss on the scale.

Give Your Liver a Vacation

The fat flush gives the liver a well-deserved vacation from its many functions. The liver synthesizes and normalizes blood protein, stores glycogen, normalizes blood fats, and manufactures bile to digest dietary fats and oils. It detoxifies the blood from the chemicals, drugs, and bacteria of all types. A liver clogged with poisons or excess fats cannot perform its essential duties.

The Fat Flush Program

The foods to be consumed for breakfast, lunch, and dinner are from the following food groups only. The list is restricted to whole natural foods eaten without salt, spices, vinegar, mustards, or herbs. These seasonings can create water retention and yeast infections. The Two-Week Fat Flush can help diminish these problems as well, so you will find the food choices pure and simple:

	The Fat Flush Protocol
Oil	1 tablespoon twice daily. Select organic high-lignan flaxseed oil for its high omega-3 metabolic-raising potential.
Lean Protein	(up to 8 ounces per day) All varieties of fish, lean beef, veal, lamb, skinless chicken, turkey, and egg whites. Vegetarians can substitute tempeh and high-protein powders with negligible carbohydrate content.
Vegetables	Low glycemic, unlimited raw, or steamed. Choose from high-fiber selections: asparagus, green beans, broccoli, brussels sprouts, cabbage, cauliflower, Chinese cabbage, cucumbers, eggplant, escarole, lettuce, okra, onions, parsley, green and red bell peppers, radishes, mung bean sprouts, tomatoes, watercress, zucchini, yellow squash, water chestnuts, bamboo shoots, garlic.
Fruits	2 whole portions daily. Choose from 1 small apple, ½ grapefruit, 1 small orange, 2 medium plums, 6 large strawberries, 10 large cherries, 1 nectarine, 1 peach.

	The Fat Flush Protocol, continued
Fruits, continued	While many other fruits are available, these choices produce the best results because they are lower on the glycemic index and so help to keep your blood sugar levels even.
Long Life Cocktail	(to increase elimination) 1 teaspoon of powdered psyllium husks in 8 ounces unsweetened cranberry juice or cranberry juice sweetened with grape concentrate (available in health food stores), taken when you wake up and before bedtime. (Metamucil is a popular brand available in most pharmacies.)

Besides the Daily Diet

- With or between meals: Drink an eight-ounce cup of hot water with juice of ½ lemon twice a day to assist kidney and liver elimination.

- Breakfast and dinner: Take supplements rich in fat-burning GLA. Choose from plain GLA supplement (90 mg.) and take 2 capsules twice daily, or choose evening primrose oil (500 mg.) and take 4 capsules twice daily.

- Take a balanced multivitamin and mineral supplement.

- Take a balanced fat-burning supplement containing liptrophic factors such as choline, methionine, inositol, 1-carnitine, and lipase.

- Drink an additional 6 glasses of pure room-temperature water per day. Room temperature is best for digestion because extremely hot or extra cold or iced drinks depress gastric juices.

- Cranberry juice contains several digestive enzymes not found in other foods. To make cranberry juice yourself, here's a simple recipe: Put 1 pound of fresh cranberries into a large saucepan. Add 5 cups of water. Boil until all berries pop. Strain juice and add a touch of grape concentrate to take the edge off the tartness. Brave souls can take it straight.

- Additional water will assist in diluting the increased body wastes from the detoxification process. Spring water or filtered water is the preferred source. Distilled water is not recommended because it can leach minerals, notably calcium, from the body and can result in a weakened heart muscle. The water should be taken consistently throughout the day, but avoid drinking huge amounts during meals so that digestive juices are not diluted. Remember that adequate amounts of water are essential to weight loss.

- Metabolizing stored fat into energy for the body is the liver's most important function. This water flush will allow the liver to operate at its best and speed up its metabolic removal of stored fats, resulting in healthy weight loss.

Detox While Dieting

Weight loss must always accompany a detoxification program. Body fat stores environmental toxins from chemicals and pesticides in food, air, and water as well as PCBs and auto exhaust. Fat can be burned off by eating the proper foods and exercising, but the toxins are generally not burned in the usual weight-loss regimen. Unburned poisons often relocate from the shrinking fat reserves to the bloodstream, organs, and tissues, causing discomfort such as headaches and nausea. Therefore, it is imperative to deal with these toxins while dieting. My Two-Week Fat Flush program does this very effectively by increasing oil, water, and exercise.

There is a twofold reason for taking the daily two tablespoons of oil:

1. Oil has metabolic-increasing power, and

2. Oil attracts the oil-soluble poisons that have been lodged in the fatty tissues of the body and carries them out of the system for elimination.

Daily Exercise

Especially important at this time is daily moderate aerobic exercise for at least twenty to thirty minutes to keep the released toxins moving.

The Water Connection

Since water is the most natural and effective diluting agent, it is important that it be used therapeutically for cleansing. Drinking any other liquids, such as coffee, tea (even herbal teas), soft drinks, diet drinks, carbonated water, mineral water, or unsweetened fruit juices, is not recommended at this time. All of these beverages contain some type of substance that must go through a digestive process. This is exactly what you don't want.

- Drinking water before a meal takes the edge off the appetite.

- Water ensures normal bowel and kidney function to rid the body of wastes as well as stored fat.

- Drinking water alleviates fluid retention, since only when the body gets plenty of water will it release the stored water.

- Water gets rid of excess salt.

- Water helps plump the skin and prevents dehydration.

- Water helps to prevent the sagging skin conditions that often follow weight loss.

Adequate amounts of water will help the kidneys filter their waste products so the liver can begin to metabolize its own waste products without having to do the kidneys' work.

Putting It All Together

A sample day from a client's diet diary on the Fat Flush Program looks like this:

	Sample Day Fat Flush Program
Upon Arising	Long Life Cocktail
	30-minute brisk walk
Before Breakfast	8 ounces hot water with lemon juice
Breakfast	Egg white omelet with mushrooms and onions
	2 90-mg. GLA capsules
	Multivitamin/mineral tablet(s)
	Fat burner supplement(s)
	8 ounces water
Midmorning	½ grapefruit
20 Minutes before Lunch	1 eight-ounce glass water
Lunch	4 ounces broiled swordfish with parsley and garlic
	Large green leafy salad with chives, sprouts, shredded cabbage, and water chestnuts
	1 tablespoon flaxseed oil
	1 eight-ounce glass water
Midafternoon	2 eight-ounce glasses water
4:00 P.M.	2 plums or 1 peach
20 Minutes before Dinner	1 eight-ounce glass water
Dinner	4 ounces baked chicken with tomatoes and onions
	4 ounces steamed asparagus
	Raw cucumber- and radish-slice salad
	1 tablespoon flaxseed oil
	Fat burner supplement(s)
	2 90-mg. GLA capsules
	8 ounces hot water with lemon juice
Midevening	Long Life Cocktail

What It Means to You

You can use this example as a basic menu guide. Just substitute foods from the same food groups for daily variety. The time frame for the Long Life Cocktail, hot water with lemon, GLA, multivitamin/mineral supplementation, and fat burner can remain approximately the same as provided in the sample guide. You can change the fluid intake to suit your schedule if that is more convenient, of course.

A Gentle Reminder: Especially for This Two-Week Period

No herbs, spices, vinegar, mustard, or soy sauce

No trans fats

No alcohol

No sugar

No oils or fats of any kind other than the daily salad oil and the good-fat supplements

No grains, bread, cereal, or starch vegetables such as beans, potatoes, corn, parsnips, carrots, peas, pumpkin, or acorn or butternut squash

No egg yolks or dairy products such as milk or cheese

Seasonal Tune-Up

This two-week cleansing diet is a marvelous body tune-up. You may want to consider doing this cleanse four times a year right before the seasons change. My patients usually take the first two weeks of January, April, July, and October to get back on track and lose their fat. Now you are ready for the next step.

For your convenience, there is now a Fat Flush Kit available; see Resources under Uni Key.

Selected References

Abraham, G. "Magnesium Deficiency in Premenstrual Tension." *Magnes Bull* 4 (1982): 68.

Abraham, G. E., and G. Harinder. "A Total Dietary Program Emphasizing Magnesium Instead of Calcium: Effect on the Mineral Density of Calcaneous Bone in Postmenopausal Women on Hormonal Therapy." *Journal of Reproductive Medicine* 35, no. 5 (May 1990).

Adlercreutz, H. "Lignans and Phytoestrogens Possible Preventive Role in Cancer." *Gastrointestinal Research* 14 (1988): 165–76.

———. "Diet and Urinary Excretion of Lignans in Female Subjects." *Medical Biology* 59 (1981): 259–61.

———. "Phytoestrogens: Epidemiology and a Possible Role in Cancer Protection." *Environmental Health Perspectives* 103, suppl. 7 (October 1995): 103–8.

———. "Dietary Phyto-Estrogens and the Menopause in Japan." *Lancet* 339 (May 16, 1992): 1233.

Anderson, K. E., and A. Kappas. "Dietary Regulation of Cytochrome P450." *Annual Review of Nutrition* 11 (1991): 141–67.

Anderson, R., and W. Wolf. "Compositional Changes in Trypsin Inhibitors, Phytic Acid, Saponins and Isoflavones Related to Soybean Processing." *Journal of Nutrition* 125, suppl. (1995): 581S–588S.

Arafat, E. S., and J. T. Hargrove. "Sedative and Hypnotic Effects of Oral Administration of Micronized Progesterone May Be Mediated Through Its Metabolites." *American Journal of Obstetrics and Gynecology* 159 (1988): 1203–9.

Arjmandi, B. H., et al. "Dietary Soybean Prevents Bone Loss in an Ovariectomized Rat Model of Osteoporosis." *Journal of Nutrition* 126 (1996): 161–67.

Atkins, R. C. *Dr. Atkins' Vita-Nutrient Solution.* New York: Simon & Schuster, 1998.

Aufrere, M. B., et al. "Progesterone: An Overview and Recent Advances." *Journal of Pharmaceutical Science* 65 (1976): 783.

Bailey, H., "GH3: Will It Keep You Young Longer?" New York: Bantam Books, 1977.

Bakan, R., "The Role of Zinc in Anorexia Nervosa: Etiology and Treatment." *Medical Hypotheses* 5 (1979).

Balch, J. F., and P. A. Balch. *Prescriptions for Nutritional Healing.* 2d ed. Garden City Park, NY: Avery, 1997.

Beattie, J. H., and H. S. Peace. "The Influence of a Low Boron Diet and Boron Supplementation on Bone Major Mineral and Sex Steroid Metabolism in a Post-Menopausal Women." *British Journal of Nutrition* (1993), 871–84.

Becker, R. O. "Fields: What You Can Do, How to Protect Yourself From the Possible Effects." *East/West* (May 1990).

Begoun, P., *Don't Go to the Cosmetics Counter Without Me.* Tukwila, WA: Beginning Press, 1991.

Beinfield, H., and E. Korngold. *Between Heaven and Earth: A Guide to Chinese Medicine.* New York: Ballantine, 1991.

Benson, H., et al. "Mind over Maladies: Can Yoga, Prayer, and Meditation Be Adapted for Managed Care?" *Hospital Health Network* 70, no. 8 (April 20, 1996): 26–27.

Bergkvist, L., et al. "The Risk of Breast Cancer After Estrogen and Estrogen-Progestin Replacement." *New England Journal of Medicine* 321, no. 5 (August 3, 1989): 293–97.

Bergner, P. "Chinese Kidney Tonics and Osteoporosis." *Medical Herbalism* 6, no. 2 (summer 1994): 1, 14.

———. *The Healing Power of Minerals, Special Nutrients, and Trace Elements.* Rocklin, CA: Prima Publishing, 1997.

Birdsall, T. C. "Gastrointestinal Candidiasis: Fact or Fiction?" *Alternative Medicine Review* 2, no. 5 (1997): 346–54.

Bland, J. S., et al. "A Medical Food Supplemented Detoxification Program in the Management of Chronic Health Problems." *Alternative Therapies in Health and Medicine* 5 (1995): 62–71.

Blaser, M. J. "The Bacteria Behind Ulcers." *Scientific American* (February 1996), 104–7.

Bradlow, H. L., et al. "Long-Term Responses of Women to Indole-3-Carbinol or a High Fiber Diet." *Cancer Epidemiol Biomarkers Prevention* 3, no. 7 (October–November 1994): 591–95.

Bremner, I. "Manifestations of Copper Excess." *American Journal of Clinical Nutrition* 67, suppl. (1998): 1069S–1073S.

"Broccoli Sprouts to Provide Cancer Protection." *Proceedings of the National Academy of Sciences* 94 (1997): 10367–72.

Brown, L. M. "Hair Dye Use in White Men and Risk of Multiple Myeloma." *American Journal of Public Health* 82, no. 12 (December 1992).

Bruner, A. B., et al. "Randomized Study of Cognitive Effects of Iron Supplementation in Non-Anaemic Iron-Deficient Adolescent Girls." *Lancet* 348 (October 12, 1996).

Burke, G. L. "The Potential Use of a Dietary Soy Supplement as Postmenopausal Hormone Replacement Therapy." Second International Symposium on the Role of Soy in Preventing and Treating Chronic Disease, Brussels, Belgium, 1996.

Businco, L., et al. "Allergenicity and Nutritional Adequacy of Soy Protein Formulas." *Journal of Pediatrics* 121 (1992): S21–S28.

Cantor, K. P., et al. "Hair Dye Use and the Risk of Leukemia and Lymphoma." *American Journal of Public Health* 78, no. 5 (May 1988).

Casper, R. "A Double-Blind Trial of Evening Primrose Oil in Premenstrual Syndrome." Second International Symposium on PMS, Kiawah Island, SC: September 1987.

Casten, D. L. *Breast Cancer: Poisons, Profits, and Prevention.* Monroe, ME: Common Courage Press, 1996.

Chakmakjian, Z., C. Higgins, and G. Abraham. "The Effect of a Nutritional Supplement, Optivite for Women, on Premenstrual Tension Syndrome: Effect of Symptomatology, Using a Double-Blind Crossover Design." *Journal of Applied Nutrition* 37 (1985): 12.

Chan, D., et al. "Regulation of Procollagen Synthesis and Processing During Ascorbate-Induced Extracellular Matrix Accumulation In-vitro." *Biochemistry Journal* 269 (1990): 175–81.

Choi, P., and P. Salmon. "Stress Responsivity in Exercisers and Non-Exercisers During Different Phases of the Menstrual Cycle." *Social Science & Medicine* 41 (1995): 769.

Chou, T. "Wake Up and Smell the Coffee: Caffeine, Coffee, and the Medical Consequences." *Western Journal of Medicine* 157, no. 5 (November 1992): 544–53.

Chuong, C. J., and E. B. Dawson. "Zinc and Copper Levels in Premenstrual Syndrome." *Fertility and Sterility* 62, no. 2 (August 1994): 313–20.

Colborn, Theo, et al. *Our Stolen Future.* New York: Penguin Books, 1997.

Colditz, G. A., et al. "The Use of Estrogens and Progestins and the Risk of Breast Cancer in Postmenopausal Women." *New England Journal of Medicine* 332, no. 24 (June 15, 1995).

Conway, P., and X. Wiang. "The Role of Probiotics and Indigestible Carbohydrates in Intestinal Health." *International Clinic of Nutrition* (July 1998).

Cowan, L. D., et al. "Breast Cancer Incidence in Women with a History of Progesterone Deficiency." *American Journal of Epidemiology* 114, no. 2 (1981): 209–17.

Cramer, D. W. "Ovarian Cancer and Talc: A Case-Control Study." *Cancer* (July 15, 1982).

Christy, C. "Vitamin E in Menopause: Preliminary Report of Experimental and Clinical Study." *American Journal of Obstetrics and Gynecology* 50 (1945): 84–87.

Cummings, R. G., et al. "Calcium Intake and Fracture Risks: Results from the Study of Osteoporosis Fractures." *American Journal of Epidemiology* 145 (1997): 926–34.

Cummings, S., et al. "Risk Factors for Hip Fracture in White Women." *New England Journal of Medicine* 332 (1997): 767–73.

Cummings, S., et al. "Bone Density at Various Sites Is Predictive of Hip Fractures." *Lancet* 341 (1993): 72–75.

Dalton, K. "The Aetiology of Premenstrual Syndrome Is with the Progesterone Receptors." *Medical Hypotheses* 31 (1987): 321–27.

———. "Erythema Multiforme Associated with Menstruation." *Journal of the Royal Society of Medicine* 78 (1985): 787–88.

———. "Influence of Menstruation on Glaucoma." *British Journal of Ophthalmology* 51, no. 10 (1987): 692–95.

———. *Premenstrual Syndrome*. London: Heinemann, 1964.

———. *The Premenstrual Syndrome and Progesterone Therapy*. 2d ed. London: Heinemann, 1984.

Darr, D., et al. "Topical Vitamin C Protects Porcine Skin from Ultraviolet Radiation–Induced Damage." *British Journal of Dermatology* 127, no. 3 (1992): 247–53.

Davis, D. L., et al. "Medical Hypothesis: Xenoestrogens as Preventable Causes of Breast Cancer." *Environmental Health Perspectives* 101, no. 5 (October 1993): 372–77.

Daweron, C. T., and M. D. Harrison. "Mechanisms for Protection Against Copper Toxicity." *American Journal of Clinical Nutrition* 67, suppl. (1998): 1091S–1097S.

Dennerstein, L., et al. "Progesterone and the Premenstrual Syndrome: A Double-Blind Crossover Trial." *British Medical Journal* 290 (1985): 1017–21.

Denollet, J. "Enhancing Emotional Well-Being by Comprehensive Rehabilitation in Patients with Coronary Heart Disease." *European Heart Journal* 16, no. 8 (August 1995): 1070–78.

Dewsilly, E., et al. "Breast Cancer and Organochlorines." *Lancet* (December 17, 1994).

Dillon, K. M., et al. "Positive Emotional States and Enhancement of the Immune System." *International Journal of Psychiatry in Medicine* 15, no. 1 (1985–86): 13–17.

"Dioxin via Skin: A Hazard at Low Doses?" *Science News* (March 4, 1989).

Eaton, B., and M. Konner. "Paleolithic Nutrition: A Consideration of Its Nature and Current Implications." *New England Journal of Medicine* 312, no. 5 (January 31, 1985): 283–89.

Ekborn, A., et al. "DDT and Testicular Cancer." *Lancet* (February 24, 1996).

Espiritu, R. C., et al. "Low Illumination Experienced by San Diego Adults: Association with Atypical Depressive Symptoms." *Biological Psychiatry* 35 (1994): 403–7.

Etcoff, Nancy L. *Survival of the Prettiest: The Science of Beauty*. New York: Doubleday, 1999.

Faclelmann, K. A. "Mixed News on Hair Dyes and Cancer Risk." *Science News* 145 (February 1994).

Fallon, S. W., and M. G. Enig. "Soy Products for Dairy Products? Not So Fast." *Health Freedom News* (September 1995).

Fiatarone, M. A., et al. "A Randomized Controlled Trial of Exercise and Nutrition for Physical Frailty in the Oldest Old." *New England Journal of Medicine* 330 (1994): 1769–75.

Folingstad, A. H. "Estriol: The Forgotten Estrogen?" *Journal of the American Medical Association* 239, no. 1 (January 2, 1978): 29–30.

Franceschi, S., et al. "Tomatoes and Risk of Digestive-Tract Cancers." *International Journal of Cancer* 59 (1994): 181–84.

Friedenwald, J., and S. Morrison. "Food Allergy in Its Relation to Gastrointestinal Disorders." *American Journal of Digestive Diseases and Nutrition* 5, no. 1 (1934): 100–103.

Frontera, W. R., et al. "Strength Conditioning in Older Men: Skeletal Muscle Hypertrophy and Improved Function." *Journal of Applied Physiology* 64 (1988): 1038–44.

Fuchs, N., *The Nutrition Detective*. San Francisco: Jeremy Tarcher, 1978.

Gambrell, R. "Update on Hormone Replacement Therapy." *American Family Physician* 46 (1992): 87S–96S.

Gannon, L. "The Potential Role of Exercise in the Alleviation of Menstrual Disorders and Menopausal Symptoms: A Theoretical Synthesis of Recent Research." *Women & Health* 14 (1988): 105.

Ginsberg, Jean. "Environmental Oestrogens." *Lancet* (January 29, 1994).

Gittleman, A. L. *Before the Change: Taking Charge of Your Perimenopause*. San Francisco: HarperSanFrancisco, 1998.

———. *Beyond Pritikin*. New York: Bantam, 1988.

———. *Super Nutrition for Menopause*. New York: Avery, 1998.

———. *Super Nutrition for Women*. New York: Bantam, 1991.

———. *Your Body Knows Best*. New York: Pocket Books, 1996.

Goei, G., and J. Ralston. "Dietary Patterns of Patients with Premenstrual Tension." *Journal of Applied Nutrition* 34 (1982): 4.

Goodale, A. Dormar, and H. Benson. "Alleviation of Premenstrual Syndrome Symptoms with the Relaxation Response." *Obstetrics and Gynecology* 75, no. 4 (April 1990): 649–89.

Goodman, M., et al. "Association of Soy and Fiber Consumption with the Risk of Endometrial Cancer." *American Journal of Epidemiology* 146, no. 4 (1997): 294–306.

Grant, E. *The Bitter Pill: How Safe Is the Perfect Contraceptive?* London: Elm Tree Books, 1985.

Haas, E. M. *Staying Healthy with the Seasons*. Millbrae, CA: Celestial Arts, 1981.

Halperin, E. C., et al. "A Double Blind, Randomized, Prospective Trial to Evaluate Topical Vitamin C Solution for the Prevention of Radiation

Dermatitis." *International Journal of Radiation Oncology Biology Physics* 26, no. 3 (1993): 413–16.

Hargrove, J. et al. "Menopausal Hormone Replacement Therapy with Continuous Daily Oral Micronized Estradiol and Progesterone." *Obstetrics and Gynecology* 73, no. 4 (1989): 606–12.

Harris, S., and B. Dawson-Hughes. "Caffeine and Bone Loss in Healthy Postmenopausal Women." *American Journal of Clinical Nutrition* 60 (1994): 573–78.

Hata, R., et al. "L-Ascorbic Acid 2-Phosphate Stimulates Collagen Accumulation, Cell Proliferation, and Formation of a Three-Dimensional Tissuelike Substance by Skin Fibroblasts." *Journal of Cellular Physiology* 138 (1989): 8–16.

Hata, R., et al. "Regulation of Collagen Metabolism and Cell Growth by Epidermal Growth Factor and Ascorbate in Cultured Human Skin Fibroblasts." *European Journal of Biochemistry* 173 (1988): 261–67.

Hayashi, A., et al. "Partial Characterization of a Unique 84-kDa Polypeptide Stimulated by Ascorbic Acid in Skin Fibroblasts." *Archives of Dermatological Research* 287 (1995): 310–14.

Henriksson, A. E. K., et al., "Small Intestinal Bacterial Overgrowth in Patients with Rheumatoid Arthritis." *Annals of Rheumatic Diseases* 52 (1993): 503–10.

Herman-Giddens, M. E., et al. "Secondary Sexual Characteristics and Menses in Young Girls Seen in Office Practice: A Study From the Pediatric Research in Office Settings." *Network Pediatrics* 99, no. 4 (1997): 505–12.

Hobbs, C. *Usnea: The Herbal Antibiotic.* Capitola, CA: Botanica Press, 1990.

Holden, J. M., et al. "Zinc and Copper in Self-Selected Diets." *Journal of the American Dietetic Association* 75 (July 1979): 23–28.

Houglum, K. P., D. A. Brenner, and M. Chojkier. "Ascorbic Acid Stimulation of Collagen Biosynthesis Independent of Hydroxylation." *American Journal of Clinical Nutrition* 54 (1991): 1141S–1143S.

"How to Avoid Pesticides," *The Nutrition Action Health Letter* 24 (5), June 1997: 1, 4–7

Hudson, T., and L. Standish. "Clinical and Endocrinological Effects of a Menopausal Botanical Formula." *Journal of Naturopathic Medicine* 7, no. 1 (1997): 73–77.

Huebner, A. "Healing Cancer with Electricity." *East/West* (May 1990).

Ivker, R. S. *Sinus Survival: The Holistic Medical Treatment for Allergies, Asthma, Bronchitis, Colds, and Sinusitis.* New York: G. P. Putnam's Sons, 1995.

Jacob, S. W., R. M. Lawrence, and M. Zucker. *The Miracle of MSM: The Natural Solution for Pain.* New York: G. P. Putnam's Sons, 1999.

Jeffers, S., *Feel the Fear . . . and Beyond.* New York: Random House, 1998.

Jenkins, D. J. A., et al. "Glycemic Index of Foods: A Physiological Basis for Carbohydrate Exchange." *The American Journal of Clinical Nutrition* 34 (March 1981): 362–66.

Jensen, B. *Tissue Cleansing Through Bowel Management.* Escondido, CA: Bernard Jensen, 1980.

Kandarkar, S. V., and P. C. Reade. "The Effect of Topical Vitamin C on Palatal Oral Mucosal Carcinogenesis Using 4-Nitroquinoline-1-oxide." *Journal of Biological Buccale* 19, no. 3 (September 1991): 199–204.

Kellar, C., *Natural Cleaning for Your Home: 95 Pure and Simple Recipes.* Asheville, NC: Lark Books, 1998.

Kelly, G. S. "Bromelain: A Literature Review and Discussion of Its Therapeutic Applications." *Alternative Medicine Review* 1, no. 4 (1996): 243–57.

Kiel, D., et al. "Hip Fracture and the Use of Estrogens in Postmenopausal Women: The Framingham Study." *New England Journal of Medicine* 317 (1987): 1169–74.

King, A., et al. "Moderate-Intensity Exercise and Self-Rated Quality of Sleep in Older Adults: A Randomized Controlled Trial." *Journal of American Medical Association* 277 (1997): 32.

Kostyniak, P. J. "Relation of Lake Ontario Fish Consumption, Lifetime Lactation, and Parity to Breast Milk Polychlorobiphenyl and Pesticide Concentrations." *Environmental Research* 80, no. 2, pt. 2 (February 1999): S166–S174.

Lee, J. *Natural Progesterone: The Multiple Roles of a Remarkable Hormone.* Sebastopol, CA: Bill Publishing, 1995.

———. "Is Natural Progesterone the Missing Link in Osteoporosis Prevention and Treatment?" *Medical Hypotheses* 35 (1991): 316–18.

Lemon, H. "Antimammary Carcinogenic Activity of 17 Alpha-Ethinyl Estriol." *Cancer* 60 (1987): 2873–81.

———. "Pathophysiologic Consideration in the Treatment of Menopausal Patients with Estrogens: The Role of Oestriol in the Prevention of Mammary Carcinoma." *Acta Endocrinologica* 233 (1980): 217–27.

Leviton, R. "Exploring Both the Health Risks and the Medical Benefits of Electromagnetic Fields." *East/West* (May 1990).

Liener, I. E. "Implications of Antinutritional Components in Soybean Foods." *Critical Reviews in Food Science Nutrition* 34 (1994): 31–67.

Longo, D. L., and R. C. Young. "Cosmetic Tale and Ovarian Cancer." *Lancet* (August 18, 1979).

Love, S., and K. Lindsey. *Dr. Susan Love's Hormone Book.* New York: Random House, 1997.

Mann, S. S. "Defensiveness and Essential Hypertension." *Journal of Psychosomatic Research* 45, no. 2 (August 1998): 139–48.

Marcola, J. M. "Oregano, Other Essential Oils Destroy Strep Pneumonia Cells." *Townsend Letter* (August/September 1998).

Marriott, P. F., et al. "Seasonality in Panic Disorder." *Journal of Affective Disorders* 31 (1994): 75–80.

Massey, L. K., et al. "Acute Effects of Dietary Caffeine and Sucrose on Urinary Mineral Excretion of Healthy Adolescents." *Nutrition Research* 8 (1988): 1005–12.

Matkovic, K. A., et al. "Menopause and Risk Factors for Coronary Heart Disease." *New England Journal of Medicine* 321, no. 10 (September 7, 1989).

Matsen, J. *Secrets to Great Health.* North Vancouver, BC: Goodwin Books, 1998.

Matsuoka, L. Y., et al. "Chronic Sunscreen Use Decreases Circulating Concentration of 25 Hydroxyvitamin D." Department of Dermatology Medical College, April 1988.

Matsuoka, L., et al. "Chronic Sunscreen Use Decreases Circulating Concentrations of 25-hydroxvitamin D," *Archives of Dermatology* 124 (December 1988), 1802–1804.

Mauvais-Jarvis, P., et al. "Estradiol/Progesterone Interaction in Normal and Pathologic Breast Cells." *Annals New York Academy Sciences,* n.d., 152–67.

Mazariegos-Ramos, E., et al. "Consumption of Soft Drinks with Phosphoric Acid as a Risk Factor for the Development of Hypocalcemia in Children: A Case-Control Study." *Journal of Pediatrics* 126 (1995): 940–42.

Messina, M., et al. "Soy Intake and Cancer Risk: A Review of the Vitro and In Vivo Data." *Nutrition and Cancer* 21 (1994): 113–31.

Moll, S., et al. "Plasma Homocysteine Levels and Mortality in Patients with Coronary Artery Disease." *New England Journal of Medicine* 337, no. 22 (November 27, 1997): 1632–33.

Monson, N. "When the Immune System Goes Awry." *Glamour* (January 1994), 20.

Morganti, C., et al. "Strength Improvements with 1 Year of Progressive Resistance Training in Older Women." *Medical Science Sports Exercise* 2 (1995): 906.

Murad, H., and C. Wood. *Murasun Suncare Products Plus Murad Environmental Shield Antioxidant Supplement Pilot Study* (unpublished), Consumer Product Testing Co., June 17, 1996.

Naimark, B., et al. "Serum Ferritin and Heart Disease: The Effect of Moderate Exercise on Stored Iron Levels in Postmenopausal Women." *Canadian Journal of Cardiology* 12 (1996): 1253.

Nelson, M. E. *Strong Women, Stay Young.* New York: Bantam Books, 1997.

Nelson, E., et al. "Effects of High-Intensity Strength Training on Multiple Risk Factors for Osteoporotic Fractures: A Randomized Controlled Trial." *Journal of the American Medical Association* 272 (1994): 1909–14.

Nielse, F. H., et al. "Boron Enhances and Mimics Some Effects of Estrogen Therapy in Postmenopausal Women." *Journal of Trace Elements in Experimental Medicine* 5 (1992): 237–46.

Nolan, K. R. "Copper Toxicity Syndrome." *Journal of Orthomolecular Psychiatry* 12, no. 4 (1983): 270–82.

Ockerman, P., et al. "Evening Primrose Oil as a Treatment of the Premenstrual Syndrome." *Recent Advances in Clinical Research* 2 (1986): 404–5.

Pearson, D. *The Natural House Book.* New York: Simon & Schuster, 1995.

Powell-Foster, K., and J. B. Miller. "International Tables of Glycemic Index." *American Journal of Clinical Nutrition* 62 (1995): 8715–35.

Prasad, A. S., and D. Oberlas, eds. *Biochemistry of Zinc.* New York: Plenum Press, 1993.

Pratt, J., and C. Longcope. "Estriol Production Rates and Breast Cancer." *Journal of Clinical Endocrinological Metabolism* 46 (1978): 44–47.

"Premenstrual Syndrome May Be Partly Linked to a Zinc Imbalance." *Better Nutrition* (July 1996), 12.

Prior, J. C.. et al. "Spinal Bone Loss and Ovulatory Disturbances." *New England Journal of Medicine* 323, no. 18 (November 1, 1990): 1221–27.

Raloff, J. "EPA: Dioxins Are More than Carcinogens." *Science News* (September 17, 1994).

———. "EcoCancers: Do Environmental Factors Underlie a Breast Cancer Epidemic?" *Science News* 144 (July 3, 1993): 10–13.

Rapkin, A. "The Role of Serotonin in Premenstrual Syndrome." *Clinical Obstetrics and Gynecology* 84, no. 6 (1994): 1001–5.

Rennie, J. "Malignant Mimicry: False Estrogens May Cause Cancer and Lower Sperm Counts." *Scientific American* (September 1993).

Ribes, G., et al. "Effect of Fenugreek Seeds on Endocrine Pancreatic Secretions in Dogs." *Annals of Nutrition & Metabolism* 28 (1984): 37–43.

Riggs, K. M., et al. "Relation of Vitamin B_{12}, Vitamin B_6, Folate and Homocysteine to Cognate Performance in the Normative Aging Study." *American Journal of Clinical Nutrition* 63 (1996): 306–14.

Robert, L., et al." The Effect of Procyanidolic Oligomers on Vascular Permeability: A Study Using Quantitative Morphology." *Pathologie Biologie* 38 (1990): 608–16.

Rodriquez, C., et al. "Estrogen Replacement Therapy and Fatal Ovarian Cancer." *American Journal of Epidemiology* 141, no. 9 (1995): 828–35.

Rooney, O. J., et al. "A Short Review of the Relationship Between Intestinal Permeability and Inflammatory Joint Disease." *Clinical and Experimental Rheumatology* 8 (1990): 75–83.

Ryle, J. A., and H. W. Barber. "Gastric Analysis in Acne Rosacea." *Lancet* (December 11, 1920), 1195–96.

Sandstrom, B., et al. "Absorption of Zinc from Soy Protein Meals in Humans." *Journal of Nutrition* 117 (1987): 321–27.

Schauss, A., and C. Costin. *Zinc and Eating Disorders.* New Canaan, CT: Keats, 1989.

Seelig, M. "Inter-relationship of Magnesium and Estrogen in Cardiovascular and Bone Disorders, Eclampsia, Migraine, and Premenstrual Syndrome." *Journal of the American College of Nutrition* 12, no. 4 (1993).

Seely, S, and D. F. Horrobin. "Diet and Breast Cancer: The Possible Connection with Sugar Consumption." *Hypotheses* 11 (1983): 319–27.

Smart, R. C., et al. "Inhibition of 12-0-tetradecanoylphorbol-13-acetate Induction of Ornithine Decarboxylase Activity, DNA Synthesis, and Tumor Promotion in Mouse Skin by Ascorbic Acid and Ascorbyl Palmitate." *Cancer Research* 47 (1987): 6633–38.

Steventon, G. B., et al. "Xenobiotic Metabolism in Alzheimer's Disease." *Neurology* 40 (July 1990): 1095–98.

Teo, K., and S. Yuuf. "Role of Magnesium in Reducing Mortality in Acute Myocardial Infarction: A Review of the Evidence." *Drugs* 46, no. 3 (1993).

Thiele, J. J., et al. "In Vivo Exposure to Ozone Depletes Vitamins C and E and Induces Lipid Peroxidation in Epidermal Layers of Murine Skin." *Free Radical Biology Medicine* 23 (1997): 385–91.

Thomas, C. *Secrets.* Solana Beach, CA: Chela Publications, 1989.

Townsley, C. *Candida Made Simple.* Littleton, CO: LFH Publishing, 1999.

"U.S. Iron Deficiency." *Lancet* (April 5, 1997), 1002.

Vale D. "Lung Cancer." *Journal of the American Academy of Nurse Practitioners* 9, no. 3 (March 1997): 143–47.

Vakkanski L. "Magnesium May Slow Bone Loss." *Medical Tribune* (July 22, 1993).

Vance, J. *Beauty to Die For: The Cosmetic Consequence.* San Diego: ProMotion, 1998.

Vecchia, C., et al. "Coffee Consumption and Myocardial Infarction in Women." *American Journal of Epidemiology* 130, no. 3 (1989): 481–85.

Verkerk, R., et al. "Effects of Processing Conditions on Glycosinolates in Cruciferous Vegetables." *Cancer Letters* 114 (March 19, 1997): 193–94.

Vesanto, M., et al. *Becoming Vegetarian.* Summertown, TN: Book Publishing, 1995.

Virtue, D. *Divine Guidance.* Los Angeles: Renaissance Books, 1998.

Watts, N., et al. "Comparison of Oral Estrogens and Estrogens Plus Androgen on Bone Mineral Density, Menopausal Symptoms, and Lipid-Lipoprotein Profiles in Surgical Menopause." *Obstetrics and Gynecology* 85 (1995): 529–37.

Webster, P. O. "Magnesium." *American Journal of Clinical Nutrition* 45, no. 5, suppl. (1987): 1305–12.

Weed, S. *Menopausal Years.* Woodstock, NY: Ash Tree Publishing, 1992.

Westin, J. B., and E. Richter. "The Israeli Breast-Cancer Anomaly." *Annals of the New York Academy of Sciences,* n.d., 269–79.

Weyerer, S, and B. Kupfer. "Physical Exercise and Psychological Health." *Sports Medicine* 17, no. 2 (1994): 108–16.

Wilgus, H. S., et al. "Goitrogenicity of Soybeans." *Journal of Nutrition* 22 (1941): 45–52.

Willett, W. C., et al. "Intake of Trans Fatty Acids and Risk of Coronary Heart Disease Among Women." *Lancet* (March 6, 1993).

Wilson, R. *Aromatherapy: For Vibrant Health & Beauty.* Garden City, NY: Avery, 1995.

Zava, D. T., and G. Duwe. "Estrogenic and Antiproliferative Properties of Genistein and Other Flavonoids in Human Breast Cancer Cells In Vitro." *Nutrition and Cancer* 27 (1997): 31–40.

Zhang, Y., et al. "A Major Inducer of Anticarcinogenic Protective Enzymes from Broccoli: Isolation and Elucidation of Structure." *Proceedings of the National Academy of Sciences* 89 (1992): 2399–2403.

Resources

Special Product Manufacturers, Distributors, and Resources

Super G.I. Cleanse, Progesta Key, Copper-Free Multiples, Parasite Cleansers, Fat Flush Kit, Salivary Hormone Testing, Books, Tissue Mineral Analysis, and H-3 Plus

Uni Key Health Systems
P.O. Box 7168
Bozeman, MT 59771
800-888-4353
unikey@unikeyhealth.com
www.unikeyhealth.com

As a convenience for my readers and clients, Uni Key has been the main distributor of my products, books, and services over the years. They carry Super G.I. Cleanse, the high-fiber supplement I prefer with the Living Beauty Elixir—paramount to sweeping away the debris clogging your intestinal tract. Progesta Key, a natural progesterone cream I developed, so critical to women of all ages, is also available through Uni Key. Progesta Key is estrogen free, and I've formulated it with essential oils for greater penetration. Uni Key also offers a copper-free multiple that I developed specifically for women who have copper overload. Para Key and Verma Plus are two parasite cleansing products that are highly effective in eliminating uninvited guests from the system. The Fat Flush Kit can be used with the Two-Week Fat Flush discussed in the Appendix. And you may order the vitally important salivary test (a special Evalu6 Test Kit that evaluates up to six hormones) and a tissue mineral analysis as well as all of my books through Uni Key. Call for a catalog of all the latest products and ask about the exclusive H-3 Plus.

Flaxseed and Evening Primrose Oil and Capsules, The Essential Woman Oil and Capsules

Barlean's Organic Oils
4936 Lake Terrell Road
Ferndale, WA 98248
800-445-3529

I designed a formula called Essential Woman that combines high-lignan flaxseed oil and evening primrose oil to meet the unique beauty and health concerns of women of all ages. This special (and delicious-tasting) product is available in both liquid and capsules. Many perimenopausal and menopausal women use the Essential Woman for balancing hormones and substitute it for the straight flaxseed oil on the detox programs. I personally use the Barlean's Greens for the Living Beauty Elixir. This super rich concentrate of nutrients, antioxidants, and phytochemicals tastes great.

Water

Essentia MicroPure Water
24100 State Route 9 SE, Bldg. A
Woodinville, WA 98072
877-293-2239
essentiawa@ad.com
www.essentiawater.com

Essentia Water, Inc. (EWI), a privately held company based in Seattle, is the leader in the field of enhanced bottled water. The firm's leading product, Essentia Water, is the only water of its kind on the market today. While detoxifying, your body tends to become acidic. Essentia uses advanced water technologies to produce good-tasting water with increased alkalinity levels. The alkalinity pH range of Essentia is 8.8 to 9.6, while other brands of bottled water are 7.0. It also supplies essential electrolytes, such as magnesium and potassium, which are needed for detox. If you are deficient in magnesium, your liver can't eliminate the toxins effectively.

In contrast to so many bottled waters, EWI avoids the use of "source" water from springs, glaciers, mountains, and so forth, because of their inconsistencies. Instead, Essentia first purifies water to its essence through reverse osmosis, then adds nutrient minerals that are much more absorbable by the body.

Three-Stage Ceramic Filter

Doulton Water Filter
CWR
Environmental Protection Products, Inc.
100 Carney Street
Glen Cove, NY 11542
800-444-3563
516-674-3788 (fax)
RSPEI3@aol.com
Unikey@unikeyhealth.com

Magnetic Watering Conditioning

GMX International
13771 Roswell Avenue, "A"
Chico, CA 91710
909-627-5700
909-627-4411 (fax)

Herb Mail Order Companies

The following mail order companies specialize in high-quality organic (nonirradiated) fresh herbs.

Herb Pharm
P.O. Box 116
Williams, OR 97544
800-348-HERB
541-846-6262

Herb Pharm is one of the only suppliers of the herb usnea, used in autumn cleansing. This company also provides botanical extracts, organic herbs and supplements, and Ayurvedic remedies.

Herbal Magic, Inc.
P.O. Box 70
Forest Knolls, CA 94933
415-488-9488

Herbal Magic offers supplement formulas, encapsulated and tableted herbs, medicinal teas, herbal teas, nutritional supplements, and children's remedies.

Blessed Herbs
109 Barre Plains Road
Oakham, MA 01068
800-489-4372
508-882-3839

Blessed Herbs carries botanicals in bulk, prepackaged herbs in smaller quantities, herbal tea bags, herbal tea blends, encapsulated wildcrafted herbs, poultice power, beehive products, herbal oils and salves, essiac formula, single herbal extracts, liquid herbal virtue formulas, aromatherapy formula oils, herbal soaps, culinary herbs and spices, books about herbs, and herbal equipment.

Aromatherapy

The following mail order companies specialize in high-quality aromatherapy products.

Aroma Vera
5901 Rodeo Road
Los Angeles, CA 90016-4312
800-669-9514
310-280-0407
   Aroma Vera offers essential oils; carrier oils; diffusers and lamps; unscented skin and body care products.

Aura Cacia
101 Paymaster
Weaverville, CA 96093
303-449-8137
   Aura Cacia provides a full line of cruelty-free personal care products, bath products, more than eighty essential oils and fragrances, soap, massage products, potpourri, candles, incense, and aromatherapy.

Original Swiss Aromatics
P.O. Box 6842
San Rafael, CA 94903
415-459-3998
   Original Swiss Aromatics offers essential oils, diffusers and lamps, and clays.

Prima Fleur Botanicals
1525 East Francisco Boulevard, Suite 16
San Rafael, CA 94901
415-455-0957
   Prima Fleur Botanicals carry a variety of unique essential oils (one-ounce minimum purchase).

Santa Fe Fragrance
P.O. Box 282
Santa Fe, NM 87504
505-473-1717

Santa Fe Fragrance provides essential oils (bulk and small quantities), exotic rare absolutes for perfumes and colognes, carrier oils, sea salts, clays, botanical cosmetic and toiletry ingredients.

Lifetree Aromatix
3949 Longridge Avenue
Sherman Oaks, CA 91423
818-986-0594

Lifetree Aromatix carries essential oils.

Homeopathy

Botanical Alchemy
P.O. Box 968
Ashland, OR 97520
800-990-2737
botanicalalchemy@botanicalalchemy.com

Botanical Alchemy is a small Oregon company with proprietary flower essence blends. This synergistic blending creates remedies with greater potency and balance than standard single-flower formulas. Botanical Alchemy uses only organic and wildcrafted flowers gathered from around the world. Formerly available exclusively through practitioners, these remarkable products can now be ordered directly.

Transformational Workshops and Consultations

Coming Alive! workshop
Christina Thomas-Fraser
991-C Lomas Santa Fe Dr.

PMB 470

Solana Beach, CA 92075

760-632-2670 (phone)

760-632-2551 (fax)

ctfraser@primenet.com

The work of Christina Thomas-Fraser is profoundly healing and life changing. Its primary focus is the clearing of emotional blockages, using BodhiSoul™ Breathwork, a safe, gentle form of rebirthing. Like me, you may find Christina's unique work a tremendous benefit, particularly if you want to change the unwanted patterns in your life, learn how to manage your emotions without shutting down or losing control, take off the "mask" and become more authentic, tap into the clarity, direction, and power of your soul, and rekindle your dreams and zest for life. As you become renewed and transformed from within, inner harmony and well being will emanate through to your physical beauty.

Through Nature's Beauty

899 South Lucerne Boulevard

Los Angeles, CA 90005

323-931-2626

Over the years, I've worked personally with Jennifer Butler, owner of Through Nature's Beauty. Thanks to her unique way of achieving color and style harmony for her clients, Jennifer was the first to tell me I was a "dramatic spring"—which made a huge difference in my wardrobe. With over ten years in the fashion industry and after years of study with Suzanne Caygill, founder of the four-season color-harmony theory, Jennifer has created a system of personalized design and color analysis. She draws upon a 4,000-swatch color system, allowing her clients to express their true selves in harmony with their surroundings. The result is a more beautiful and more harmonious individual, whether the client is male or female.

Additional Helpful Information

Contacting Me (I'd Love to Hear from you!)

On the Web

If you want to read my recent articles that have appeared in a variety of national publications, see a listing of all my books, or obtain a schedule of my upcoming events, just hop on the Web and visit my site: www.annlouise.com. Or email me at gittleman@mindspring.com.

Key to Health Foundation
P.O. Box 882
Bozeman, MT 59771
gittleman@mindspring.com

Dedicating my career to women's health has been tremendously rewarding. But I wanted to help women even more, so I began searching for a venue to accomplish that deep-seated desire. I knew that if women partnered together, we could promote the health of women to even higher levels. And that prompted me to create a nonprofit organization called Key to Health.

Key to Health is committed to bettering women's health and well-being by supporting specific organizations that parallel its mission, principles, and holistic philosophy. Through these combined, dedicated efforts, Key to Health hopes to create a platform that will not only help and empower women at every transition of their lives, but also set in motion a nutritional revolution that will reach out to future generations as well.

If you would like to learn more about Key to Health and how you can become a partner in my quest to promote woman's health, please write or e-mail for an introductory packet.

Nutrition and Health Organizations

American Menopause Foundation
The Empire State Building
350 Fifth Avenue, Suite 2822
New York, NY 10118

212-714-2398

212-714-1252 (fax)

menopause@earthlink.net

The American Menopause Foundation is the only independent, not-for-profit organization dedicated to providing support and assistance on all issues concerning the change of life. The network of volunteer support groups serves as a resource for women, families, organizations, and corporations. The foundation's newsletter, literature, and educational programs provide the latest information on scientific research and other pertinent facts related to the change of life.

Price-Pottenger Nutrition Foundation

P.O. Box 2614

La Mesa, CA 91943-2614

619-574-7763

619-547-1314 (fax)

info@price-pottenger.org

The Price-Pottenger Nutrition Foundation is a not-for-profit, tax-exempt educational organization dedicated to the promotion of enhanced health through awareness of ecology, lifestyle, and healthy food production for sound nutrition. At its core are the landmark works of Drs. Weston A. Price and Francis M. Pottenger Jr., pioneers in modern research.

The Name Brand Shopping List for the Living Beauty Detox Diet

For your convenience I have provided a name brand shopping list for the Living Beauty Detox Diet program and maintenance plan. Most of these foods can be found in your health food store, food co-op, or organic section of the supermarket. For those items that are more difficult to obtain, I have provided telephone numbers.

Super Green Food

Barlean's Greens

Greens +

ProGreens

Greens Today

Earth Source Greens and More

Kyo-Greens

Green Vibrant

High Fiber Supplement

Super GI Cleanse, 800-888-4353 (Uni Key Health Systems)

Super GI Cleanse is especially formulated for seasonal cleansing. The herbs, digestive enzymes and intestinal flora target the liver, kidneys, colon, and lymph.

Organic Dairy

Nancy's

Horizon

Cascadian Farms

Organic Protein

Belle Brook Farms, 800-830-2354

Shelton Farms

Harmony Farms

Foster Farms

Young Farms

Coleman Natural Beef

Mori-Nu tofu

White Wave tofu

The Name Brand Shopping List for Living Beauty Products

For your convenience I have provided a name brand shopping list for health and beauty products that are mentioned in this book. Most of these products can be found in your health food store, cosmetics section of large department stores, drugstores, and pharmacies. For those items that are more difficult to obtain, I have provided telephone numbers.

Topical Vitamin C

Cellex-C

Skin Ceuticals

C-Esta

ShiKai Dermaceutical Formulations

Jason's Topical C

Orange Daily 10% Topical Serum

Murad's Topical Vitamin C Antioxidant

Retinol Topicals

Estee Lauder's Diminish

Avon Anew Retinol Recovery Complex PM Treatment

Special Collagen Boosters

Estee Lauder's Resilience Lift

Brown Spots

Dermalogica's Pigment Relief, 800-831-5150

Enrich International Fade Crème, 801-226-2600

Nail Moisturizer

SuperLan, 917-352-7331

SuperLan also relieves dry, cracked lips, heels, elbows, and nipples dried from breast-feeding.

Varicose Veins

Venastat

Just Natural's Horse-Chestnut & Yarrow Leg and Vein Crème, 802-362-2400

Natural Breast Augmentation

Erdic, 877-495-9511 or contact www.original-erdic.com

After gaining more fullness and firmness I, too, became a believer.

Eczema

Aveeno (colloidal oatmeal products)

Scars

Mederma

Clinicel

ReJuveness

These products are available through drugstores or the Internet.

Natural Progesterone Creams

Angel Care, from Angel Care

Bio Balance, from Garon Pharmaceuticals

Equilibrium, from Equilibrium Lab

Femme Naturale, from Sarati International

NatraGest, from Broadmoore Labs

OstaDerm, from Bezwecken

PhytoGest, from Karuna Corporation

Pro-Alo, from HealthWatchers

ProBalance, from Springboard

Pro-G, from TriMedica

Pro-Gest, from Professional & Technical Services

Progesta Key

(Progesta Key is my own formulation, which includes vitamin E, evening primrose oil, yarrow, and lavender extract. It comes in a unique pump style container, which dispenses the recommended amount of cream with an easy stroke of the pump. I developed this to be one of the most effective and reasonably priced natural progesterone creams on the market today.)

The Name Brand Shopping List for Living Beauty Miscellaneous Products

Chocolate

Newman's Own Organics

Sunspire Organic

Rapunzel Natural

Green & Black's, 904-825-2057

Coffee

Montana Coffee Trader

Jim's Organic Coffee

Café Mam

Produce Wash

Healthy Harvest, 203-245-2033

Natural Paints and Stains

Auro Products, 707-427-2325

Livos Plantchemistry, 505-988-9111

Household Cleansers

Amidst the many biodegradable, nontoxic cleansers available on the market, here are the ones I have personally used and recommend. Try to locate a local distributor in your area. They should be listed in the phone book or available through the Internet.

Shaklee

Amway

Young Living

Melaleuca

Index

Abraham, Guy, 22, 126, 182
aching muscles, 145
acid mantle, 117–18. *See also* aging skin
acne vulgaris, 109, 122
adrenal glands, 96–97
adrenal insufficiency, 131
adrenal stress, 96–97
affirmation, 158–61
aging skin: the acid mantle and, 117–18;
    skin care products for, 115–18; wrinkle
    busters for, 112–13, 128–29. *See also* skin
alcohol, 113
allergies, 68
almond meal mask, 132
alpha-hydroxies, 115
*Alternative Therapies in Health and
    Medicine* (Bland), 28–29
American Association of Naturopathic
    Physicians Conference (1992), 60
American Heart Association, 81
American Journal of Epidemiology (jour-
    nal), 22
American Journal of Public Health (jour-
    nal), 163
anemia, 131
anise, 83
antibiotics, 25
antioxidants (topical), 114–15
ants, 172
Archives of Dermatology (journal), 20
aromatherapy, 93–94

aromatherapy facial oil recipe, 124–25,
    130
Atkins Clinic, 143
Atkins Diet, The, 17
autoimmune diseases, 68
Autumn Detox Diet: exercises for, 92–93;
    following the, 83–84; healing tea, herbs,
    spices for, 83; protocol for, 84–85; sam-
    ple day one of, 85–86; sample day three
    of, 87–88; sample day two of, 86–87;
    supporting treatments for
    respiration/colon, 93–94
Autumn Detox Maintenance: menu plan for,
    91–92; plan for, 88–91
Autumn (Type 3): described, 78–83; deter-
    mining, 44–46, 48

Bach, Edward, 151
Bach Flower Remedies, 151–54
Bakan, R., 21
Ball, Lucille, 147
B-complex vitamins, 122
beans selection: for Autumn Detox Plan,
    90; for Spring Detox Plan, 58; for
    Summer Detox Plan, 74; for Winter
    Detox Plan, 103
beauty: eating your way to, 30–32; innate
    fascination with, 2–3; path to inner,
    149–51; self-esteem issues associated
    with, 3–4; unlocking your individual,
    10–11

beauty basic drills: cleanse, tone, and
    moisturize, 119–20; exfoliate and apply
    masks, 120; topical essential oils,
    120–21
beauty basic truths: about the acid mantle,
    117–18; about essential fatty acids, 112;
    about the sun, 110–12; about water, 119;
    about wrinkle busters, 112–13
"beauty detectors," 3
beauty routines: during the fifties and six-
    ties, 138–46; during the teens and twen-
    ties, 122–27; during the thirties and
    forties, 127–38; importance of, 108–9
Bee's Secret, 142
Before the Change (Gittleman), 22
Begoun, Paula, 116
Benbrook, Charles, 166
Benson, Herbert, 156
benzophenone, 111
Bergner, Paul, 166
Beyond Pritikin Diet, 17
Beyond Pritikin (Gittleman), 50
biodegradable cleaning products, 172–74
bioflavonoids, 124
biotin, 187
birth control pills, 20–21, 83
bladder, 95–96
Bland, Jeffrey, 15, 28, 29, 82
blotchy skin, 132–33
BodhiSoul breathwork, 150
bones: during fifties and sixties, 138; dur-
    ing teens and twenties, 126–27
Botanical Alchemy, 152
botanical alchemy emotional remedies,
    152–54
bread and grains selection: for Autumn
    Detox Plan, 90; for Winter Detox Plan,
    103
breast augmentation, 146
brittle nails, 135–36
bromium, 123
brown spots, 130–31
burdock root, 126
buttermilk mask, 132

caffeine, 36, 113
calamine lotion, 123
calcium, 22, 191–92

calcium craze, 22–23
calcium zappers, 126
Campbell, Naomi, 3
carbohydrate-free diets, 17–19
carbon dioxide, 80–81
castor oil, 127
castor oil pack, 60–61
Caygill, Suzanne, 95
chamomile tea, 128
Chanel, Coco, 108
Chinese medicine. *See* traditional Chinese
    medicine
chlordane, 171–72
chlorine, 25, 169–70
chocolate (organic), 167
choline, 187
cigarette smoking, 80, 113
cleanse, tone, and moisturize drill, 119–20
cleansing oils, 32–33, 38
Cleopatra, 3, 130
Clorox baths, 34
cockroaches, 172
coffee (organic), 167
Colburn, Theo, 9
collagen, 116
collagen loss, 129
colon, 81, 82–83
colon therapy, 94
Condemi, John J., 9
connecting breathing, 154–56
copper, 16, 37, 196–97
copper overload, 96–97, 109
cortisol, 96
cosmetics, 163–65
cosmetic surgery, 145–46
cracked lips, 135
cranberry juice, 39
Crawford, Cindy, 3
cucumber masks, 131
cytochrome P-450 enzymes, 30

dairy selection: for Autumn Detox Plan, 91;
    for Spring Detox Plan, 58; for Summer
    Detox Plan, 74; for Winter Detox Plan,
    103
dark circles, 128
Denollet, Johan, 149
depression, 141–42

dermatitis, 142
detoxing the inner: affirmation for, 158–61;
    connected breathing for, 154–56; flower
    remedies for, 151–54; importance of,
    147–49; meditation for, 156–58; path to
    healing/inner beauty, 149–51. *See also*
    Living Beauty Detox Diet
detoxing the outer: cosmetics for, 163–65;
    creating relaxing environment, 175–76;
    foods for, 166–67; household chemicals,
    171–74; household interiors, 174–75;
    importance of, 162; water, 40, 119,
    169–71. *See also* Living Beauty Detox
    Diet
diets: carbohydrate-free, 17–19; fat-free,
    14–16
digestive process: impaired, 64–65; process
    of, 65–66
Divine Guidance (Virtue), 159
dry hair, 134
dry nails, 137
dry skin, 129–30, 139–40
dull hair, 133–34
dysbiosis (leaky gut), 82

Ecclesiastes, 49
eczema, 142–43
EFAs, 198
elastin, 116
enlarged facial pores, 132
Environmental Protection Agency, 167
environmental stress, 113
essential fatty acids (EFAs), 112
essential oils, 120–21, 130
Estée Lauder, 1, 2
estrogen, 23–24, 199
estrogen dominance, 24, 29, 37, 109, 125
Etcoff, Nancy, 2, 3
exercise: for Autumn Detox Diet, 92–93;
    during Two-Week Fat Flush program,
    207; low estrogen reserves and, 126–27;
    for Spring Detox Diet, 59–60; for
    Summer Detox Diet, 75–76; for Winter
    Detox Diet, 106; wrinkles and lack of,
    113
exfoliate/apply masks drill, 120
exfoliating dead skin cells, 124
eye bright herb tea, 127

eyes: dark circles under, 128; lines under
    the, 127; puffy, 127–28; tired, 140

face-lift, 145–46
facial hair, 125, 133
facials: aromatherapy facial oil recipe for,
    124–25, 130; mayonnaise, 130. *See also*
    masks
fasting, 28–30
fat-free diets, 14–16, 113
fenugreek tea, 83, 88
fiber-rich supplement, 40
fifties' beauty routines, 138–46
flower remedies, 151–54
folic acid, 188
foods. *See* organic foods
forties' beauty routines, 127–38
freckles, 130–31
free radicals, 29, 113–14
fruits, 34, 39, 167–69
Fuchs, Nan Kathryn, 22, 23

Garland, Cedrick, 111, 112
Garland, Frank, 111, 112
garlic, 68
gastrointestinal tract, 64–66, 69, 81–82
ginger, 98
glutathione, 29, 31
Goodale, A. Dormar, 156
good intentions: additional hazards caused
    by, 24–25; of beauty/health and modern-
    day hazards, 23–24; of birth control
    pills, 20–21, 83; of calcium craze,
    22–23; of carbohydrate-free diets,
    17–19; of fat-free diets, 14–16, 113; rid-
    ding ourselves of mistaken, 25–26; of
    sunscreen, 19–20
Graham, Karen, 2
grains and bread selection: for Autumn
    Detox Plan, 90; for Winter Detox Plan,
    103
grief, 151
gums, 139

hair: dry and oily, 134; dull, 133–34; facial,
    125, 133; listed problems/solutions for,
    180; thinning, 138–39
hair dyes, 24–25, 163

hair loss, 134–35

Hampton, Aubrey, 163

Harrison, Clifton, 152

Healing Power of Mineral, Special Nutrients, and Trace Elements, The (Bergner), 166

Health & Healing (newsletter), 169

HealthComm Clincial Research Center, 29, 82

heart, 64

Hepar sulph calcarean, 123

herbs: for Autumn Detox Diet, 83; recommendations for, 34–35; for Spring Detox Diet, 52–53; for Summer Detox Diet, 67–68; for Winter Detox Diet, 98

Hippocrates, 27

hormones, 199–201

household chemicals, 171–74

household interiors, 174–75

hydrating skin, 124

hydrochloric acid, 65–67

hydrogenated oils, 122

impaired digestive tract, 64–65

inner beauty, 149–51

inositol, 186

insomnia, 140–41

insulin, 125

International Journal of Alternative and Complementary Medicine (Larsen), 111

iodine, 123

iron, 195–96

Jeffers, Susan, 159

Johns Hopkins University study, 148

Journal of Applied Nutrition (Bland), 29

Journal of Clinical Endocrinology and Metabolism (journal), 20

Journal of Reproductive Medicine (journal), 22

Kali bromatum, 123

Kennedy, Jacqueline, 25

kidney cleansing, 98

kidneys, 95–96

Kirley, George E., 203

Lancet study (1997), 33

Lancet, The (journal), 24

Langerhan's cells, 111

large intestines, 81

Larsen, Hans, 111

leaky gut (dysbiosis), 82

Lee, John, 24

Leonardo Da Vinci, 13

L-glutamine, 68, 123

lignans, 33

lines under the eyes, 127

liver: cleansing the, 131; excess toxins in, 96; necessary functions of, 31–32; Springtime supporting treatments for, 60–61

Living Beauty Alphabet of Vitamins and Minerals: described, 6, 177–78; EFAs, 198; for hair problems, 180; hormones, 199–201; minerals, 191–90; for nail problems, 180; for skin problems, 178–80; for tongue problems, 181; vitamins, 181–91

Living Beauty Cleansing Questionnaire, 40–48

Living Beauty Detox Diet: benefits of, 28; caffeine avoidance and, 36; elements of, 6; fiber-rich supplement as part of, 40; fruits as part of, 34, 39; healing teas, herbs, spices as part of, 34–35; learning the principles of, 11–12; limiting sugars in, 35–36; Living Beauty Elixir as part of, 39; protein as part of, 32, 38; protocol of, 37–40; purified water as part of, 40; for Spring, 52–57; for Summer, 67–73; to repair toxic damage, 10; vegetables as part of, 33–34, 38–39; zinc as part of, 36–37. *See also* detoxing the inner

Living Beauty Detox program: elements of, 6; mainstays of, 6–7; procedures of, 37–40; results of, 5

Living Beauty Elixir, 39, 53–54, 57, 88

Loren, Sophia, 1

Love, Medicine, and Miracles (Siegel), 156

L. plantarum bacteria, 68–69

lumphatic cleansing, 76–77

lung cancer, 80

lungs, 79

lycopene, 115

magnesium, 22, 126, 128, 192–93
manganese, 197–98
Mann, Samuel, 149
Mark Antony, 3
masks: almond meal, 132; buttermilk, 132; cucumber, 131; exfoliate/applying, 120; milk of magnesia, 124, 132; oatmeal, 130; yogurt toning, 19. *See also* facials
mayonnaise facial, 130
Medical Hypothese (journal), 21
Medical Tribune (journal), 22
meditation, 156–58
melanoma, 111
milk of magnesia mask, 124, 132
minerals, 191–90
miso, 98
Monroe, Marilyn, 3, 4
mouth corner cracks, 135
mullein, 83
Murad, Howard, 112
muscles: aching, 145; sagging, 145

nail fungus, 136–37
nails: brittle, 135–36; dry, 137; listed problems/solutions for, 180
Naparstek, Belleruth, 159
National Cancer Institute hair dye study, 24–25
National Cancer Institute survey (1992), 163
Natural Cleaning for Your Home: 95 Pure and Simple Recipes (Lark Books), 173
Natural Ingredients Dictionary Plus Ten Synthetic Cosmetic Ingredients to Avoid (Hampton), 164
nettle tea, 98
New England Journal of Medicine (journal), 21, 63
niacinamide (niacin), 185
Nutrition Action Health Letter (Center for Science in the Public Interest), 166
nuts selection: for Autumn Detox Plan, 90–91; for Winter Detox Plan, 103–5

oatmeal mask, 130
oils: critical for cleansing, 32–33; essential, 120–21, 130; hydrogenated, 122; tea tree, 123; therapeutic, 38

oily hair, 134
oily skin, 124
olive leaf extract, 144
omega-3 fatty acids, 14–15, 18
omega-6 fatty acids, 14–15
organic coffee, 167
organic foods: Detox Diet bean selections, 58, 74, 90, 103; Detox Diet grains/bread selection, 90, 103; Detox Diet nuts selection, 90–91, 103–5; Detox Diet vegetable selections, 58, 73, 89–90, 103; for detoxing the outer, 166–67; Detox Plan dairy selection, 58, 74, 91, 103; fruits, 34, 39, 167–69; vegetables, 33–34, 38–39, 167–69
organs, 49–50, 51

PABA, 186
pale skin, 131–32
panthenol, 126
pantothenic acid, 188–89
parasite infestation, 128
Peat, Raymond, 24
People magazine survey (1999), 4
pesticides, 167, 171–72
petachiae (elevated red spots), 131
pH-balanced products, 118
phosphorus, 193
Physician's Health Study (Harvard, 1996), 64
phytonutrient sources, 18
Picture of Dorian Gray, The (Wilde), 11
Pill, the, 20–21, 83
pollutant-free environment, 80–81
Porgy and Bess, 62
pregnancy mask, 142
Price, Weston A., 162
probiotic formula, 122–23
problem gums, 139
progesterone, 24, 200
progesterone deficiency, 125
protein: as detox powerhouse, 32, 38; missing in fat-free diets, 15–16
psoriasis, 143–44, 179
puffy eyes, 127–28
purified water, 40

rashes, 142
rebounding treatments (Summer Detox Diet), 76
relaxing environment, 175–76
Renova, 115, 127, 129
Rescue Remedy, 151
respiration treatments, 93–94
respiratory tract, 79–80
Retin-A, 115, 129
Retinol, 115, 129
Rodin, 10–11
"Role of Zinc in Anorexia Nervosa: Etiology and Treatment, The" (Bakan), 21
rosacea, 142

sagging muscles, 145
St. John's wort, 141
salty foods, 123
sauerkraut, 68–69
scars, 144
seafood, 123
Seasonal Affective Disorder (SAD), 78, 93, 95, 97
seasons: detox program based on, 50–52; linked to specific organs, 49–50, 51; symptoms associated with, 50
season types: determining dominant, 41, 48; Type 1: Spring, 41–43, 48; Type 2: Summer, 43–44, 48; Type 3: Autumn, 44–46, 48; Type 4: Winter, 46–47, 48
seawater rinses, 94
secondhand smoke, 80, 81
selenium, 194–95
sensitive skin, 124–25
Siegel, Bernie, 156–57
sinuses, 79–80
sixties' beauty routines, 138–46
skin: acid mantle of, 117–18; aging, 112–13, 115–18; blotchy, 132–33; drinking water and, 119; dry, 129–30, 139–40; enlarged facial pores, 132; exfoliating, 124; hydrating, 124; listing problems/solutions for, 178–80; oily, 124; pale, 131–32; as protection, 178; sensitive, 124–25
skin brushing, 77

skin cancer epidemic, 111–12
skin care products: antiaging creams, 116–18; topical antioxidant creams, 115. See also aging skin; cosmetics
skin DNA cellular structure, 113–14
small intestine, 64–65, 68
smoking: dangers of, 80; wrinkles caused by, 113
spices: for Autumn Detox Diet, 83; recommendations for, 34–35; for Spring Detox Diet, 52–53; for Summer Detox Diet, 67–68; for Winter Detox Diet, 98
spider veins, 137
split ends, 126
Spring Detox Diet: beans selection for, 58; exercise for, 59–60; protocol for, 54; sample day one for, 55; sample day three for, 56–57; sample day two for, 55–56; starchy vegetables selection for, 58; tea, herbs, spices for, 52–53
Spring Detox Maintenance: plan for, 57–58; sample menu plan for, 59
Springtime liver/gallbladder supporting treatments, 60–61
Spring (Type 1): determining, 41–43, 48; Living Beauty Detox Diet for, 52–57
starchy vegetables selection. See vegetable selection
Stein, Gertrude, 177
Stephen Paul, 150–51
stress: adrenal glands and, 96–97, 107; wrinkles and environmental, 113
stretch marks (striae), 144–45
sugars, 35–36, 122, 125
sulfur, 195
Summer Detox Diet: circulatory supporting treatments during, 76–77; exercise for, 75–76; following the, 68–69; healing tea, herbs, spices for, 67–68; protocol for, 69–70; sample day one for, 70–71; sample day three for, 72–73; sample day two for, 71–72
Summer Detox Maintenance: menu plan for, 74–75; plan for, 73–74
Summer (Type 2): described, 62–67; determining, 43–44, 48
sunlight, 97

sunscreen: choosing, 110–11; as good
   intention, 19–20
sun, the, 110–12
Super Nutrition for Menopause (Gittleman),
   22
*Survivial of the Prettiest: The Science of
   Beauty* (Etcoff), 2

talcum powder, 24
tamari, 98
tannic acid, 128
tea: for Autumn Detox Diet, 83; recommendations for, 34–35; for Spring Detox Diet,
   52–53; for Summer Detox Diet, 67–68;
   for Winter Detox Diet, 98
tea tree oil, 123
teenage year beauty routines, 122–27
"Ten Synthetic Cosmetic Ingredients to
   Avoid," 163–65
termites, 172
testosterone, 200–201
therapeutic oils, 32–33, 38
thinning hair, 138–39
thirties' beauty routines, 127–38
tired eyes, 140
tobacco smoking, 80, 113
tongue problems/solutions, 181
topical antioxidants, 114–15
topical essential oils drill, 120–21
"Total Dietary Program Emphasizing
   Magnesium Instead of Calcium, A"
   (Abraham), 22
Townsend Letter for Doctors and Patients
   (Wolverton), 174
Townsley, Cheryl, 77
toxic overload: modern-day sources of,
   23–24; results of, 7–8; sources of,
   8–10
traditional Chinese medicine: on acupuncture meridians, 40–41; on emotion of
   grief, 151; on "fire" of heart, 64; purifying program based on, 49
twenties' beauty routines, 122–27
Two-Week Fat Flush program: additional
   elements of, 205–6, 209; described, 50,
   203; detox while dieting using, 206;
   exercise during, 207; protocol for,

204–5; sample day menu for, 208; water
   during, 207
Type 1. *See* Spring: Type 1
Type 2. *See* Summer: Type 2
Type 3. *See* Autumn: Type 3
Type 4. *See* Winter: Type 4
Type D patients, 149
tyrosine, 142

USA Today, 148
usnea, 83
UVB and UVA protection, 110, 111, 115

Vale, Darla, 149
Vance, Judi, 9
varicose veins, 137–38
vegetables, 33–34, 38–39, 167–69
vegetable selection: for Autumn Detox Diet,
   89–90; for Spring Detox Diet, 58; for
   Summer Detox Diet, 73; for Winter
   Detox Diet, 103
veins: spider, 137; varicose, 137–38
Virtue, Doreen, 159
vitamin A, 2, 29, 30, 33, 115, 123, 181–82
vitamin A deficiency, 128, 129, 143
vitamin B_1 (thiamin), 183
vitamin B_2 (riboflavin), 183–84
vitamin B_6 (pyridoxine), 122, 184
vitamin B_{12}, 184–85
vitamin B complex, 182–83
vitamin C, 2, 29, 30, 114–15, 124, 129,
   189
vitamin C serum, 129
vitamin D, 33, 110, 189–90
vitamin D deficiency, 19–20, 190
vitamin E, 2, 29, 30, 33, 112, 115, 129, 190
vitamin K, 33, 191

Ward, William Arthur, 159
water: chlorine connection, 169–70; drinking purified, 40, 119; during Two-Week
   Fat Flush, 207; how to purify, 170–71
whistle lines, 135
Whitaker, Julian, 169
Wilde, Oscar, 11
Winter Detox Diet: exercise for, 106; following plan for, 98–99; protocol for, 99;

sample day one for, 99–100; sample day
    three for, 101–2; sample day two for,
    100–1; supporting treatments during,
    106–7; tea, herbs, spices for, 98
Winter Detox Maintenance: food selections
    for, 103–5; menu plan for, 105; plan for,
    102
Winter (Type 4): described, 95–97; deter-
    mining, 46–47, 48
witch hazel, 132

Wolverton, Bill, 174
Wordsworth, William, 78
wrinkle busters, 112–13, 128

yogurt toning mask, 129

zinc, 16, 21, 36–37, 122, 126, 194
zinc deficiency, 96, 109
Zone Diet, The, 17